SPRINGER PU[BLISHING]
YOUR ONE-S[TOP]
FOR ALL OF YOUR EXAM PREP NEEDS

- **BOOKS & FLASHCARDS**
- **SELF-PACED DIGITAL COURSES**
- **DIGITAL QBANKS**

Give yourself the confidence to pass your next exam with solutions that fit any stage of your study plan. Springer Publishing's ExamPrepConnect offers instant access to digital products and content created by experts that will help you ace your next certification — from comprehensive reviews to short, focused Q&A.

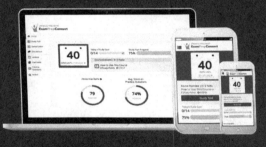

SAVE 25%
ON YOUR NEXT CERTIFICATION PREP PURCHASE WITH CODE ONESTOP25

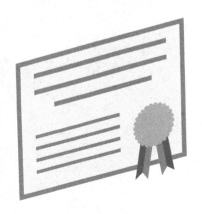

Becoming certified will help you get ahead of the competition, earn more money, and get the jobs you want. Springer Publishing can help you take the next step in your career with print and digital exam prep solutions tailored to your study style.

Learn more at Springerpub.com/examprep

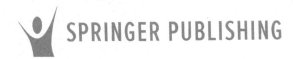

SPRINGER PUBLISHING

CDCES® Certification Practice Q&A

CDCES® Certification
Practice Q&A

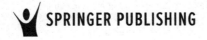
SPRINGER PUBLISHING

Springer Publishing Company, LLC
11 West 42nd Street, New York, NY 10036
www.springerpub.com

Acquisitions Editor: Elizabeth Nieginski
Compositor: diacriTech

ISBN: 9780826145819
ebook ISBN: 9780826145826
DOI: 10.1891/9780826145826

22 23 24 / 5 4 3 2 1

The author and the publisher of this Work have made every effort to use sources believed to be reliable to provide information that is accurate and compatible with the standards generally accepted at the time of publication. The author and publisher shall not be liable for any special, consequential, or exemplary damages resulting, in whole or in part, from the readers' use of, or reliance on, the information contained in this book. The publisher has no responsibility for the persistence or accuracy of URLs for external or third-party Internet websites referred to in this publication and does not guarantee that any content on such websites is, or will remain, accurate or appropriate.

Library of Congress Control Number: 2022939854

Contact sales@springerpub.com to receive discount rates on bulk purchases.

Publisher's Note: **New and used products purchased from third-party sellers are not guaranteed for quality, authenticity, or access to any included digital components.**

Printed in the United States of America by Hatteras, Inc.

Contents

Preface

Welcome to *CDCES® Certification Practice Q&A*! Congratulations on taking this important step on your journey to becoming a certified diabetes care and education specialist. This resource is based on the most recent Certification Board for Diabetes Care and Education (CBDCE) exam blueprint and was developed by experienced diabetes care and education specialists. It is designed to help you sharpen your specialty knowledge with 200 practice questions organized by exam subject area, as well as strengthen your knowledge-application and test-taking skills with a 200-question practice exam. It also includes essential information about the Certification Examination for Diabetes Care and Education Specialists® (CDCES®), including eligibility requirements, exam subject areas and question distribution, and tips for successful exam preparation.

▶ PART I: PRACTICE QUESTIONS

Part I includes three chapters based on the exam blueprint: Assessment of the Diabetes Continuum, Interventions for Diabetes Continuum, and Disease Management. Each chapter includes high-quality, exam-style questions and comprehensive answers with rationales that address both correct and incorrect answers. Part I is designed to strengthen your specialty knowledge and is formatted for ultimate studying convenience—answer the questions on each page and simply turn the page for the corresponding answers and rationales. No need to refer to the back of the book for the answers.

▶ PART II: PRACTICE EXAM

Part II includes a 200-question practice exam that aligns with the content domains and question distribution on the most recent CDCES® exam blueprint. This practice exam is designed to help you strengthen your knowledge-application and test-taking skills. Maximize your preparation and simulate the exam experience by setting aside 4 hours to complete the practice exam. Comprehensive answers and rationales that address both correct and incorrect answers are located in the chapter immediately following the practice exam.

We know life is busy, and being able to prepare for your exam efficiently and effectively is paramount. This resource will give you the tools and confidence you need to succeed. For additional exam preparation resources, including self-paced online courses, online QBanks, comprehensive review texts, and high-yield study guides, visit www.springerpub.com/examprep. Best of luck to you on your certification journey!

Introduction: CDCES® Certification Exam and Tips for Preparation

▶ ELIGIBILITY REQUIREMENTS

The Certification Examination for Diabetes Care and Education Specialists® (CDCES®) is developed and administered by the Certification Board for Diabetes Care and Education (CBDCE). To qualify to take the exam, you must meet the following requirements:

- Current, active, unrestricted license from the United States or its territories as a clinical psychologist, RN (including nurse practitioner and clinical nurse specialist), occupational therapist, optometrist, pharmacist, physical therapist, physician (MD or DO), or podiatrist;
  or
- Dietitian or dietitian nutritionist holding active registration with the Commission on Dietetic Registration, physician assistant holding active registration with the National Commission on Certification of Physician Assistants, exercise physiologist holding active certification as an American College of Sports Medicine Certified Clinical Exercise Physiologist, or health educator holding active certification as a Master Certified Health Education Specialist from the National Commission for Health Education Credentialing;
  or
- Healthcare professional with a minimum of a master's degree in social work from a U.S. college or university accredited by a nationally recognized regional accrediting body
  and
- A minimum of 2 years of professional practice experience in the discipline under which you are applying for certification
  and
- A minimum of 1,000 hours of diabetes care and education experience (accrued within 5 years before applying for certification) with a minimum of 20% (200 hours) of those hours accrued in the most recent year before application
  and
- A minimum of 15 clock-hours of continuing education activities applicable to diabetes within the 2 years before applying for certification

Qualified applicants may submit an online or paper application. Successful candidates will receive a confirmation notice with a toll-free telephone number and website address to schedule the exam within a 90-day window. The exam fee is $350; the fee for renewal of certification is $250. Refer to the CBDCE website for complete eligibility requirements, pricing, and certification information: www. cbdce.org/become-certified

▶ ABOUT THE EXAMINATION

The CDCES® exam takes 4 hours and consists of 200 multiple-choice questions with four answer options. You must select the single best answer. Only 175 questions are scored, and the remaining 25 questions are used as pretest questions. It is impossible to know which questions are scored, so be sure to answer all of the questions to the best of your ability.

See Table 1 for exam content domains and question distribution. For more detailed exam content information, refer to the exam content outline in the CBDCE *Certification for Diabetes Care and Education Specialists Handbook.*

Table 1. CDCES® Exam Content Domains and Question Distribution

Content Domain	Number of Questions (Scored)
Assessment of the Diabetes Continuum	59
Interventions for Diabetes Continuum	88
Disease Management	28

Source: Data from Certification Board for Diabetes Care and Education: *Certification for Diabetes Care and Education Specialists Handbook.* 2022. https://www.cbdce.org/documents/20123/108727/ CEHandbookCurrent.pdf/82de0066-76f3-d4ff-485f-ca670f6f83bd?t=1647012109595

▶ TIPS FOR EXAM PREPARATION

You know the old joke about how to get to Carnegie Hall—practice, practice, practice! The same is true when seeking certification. Practice and preparation are key to your success on exam day. Here are 10 tips to help you prepare:

1. Allow at least 6 months to fully prepare for the exam. Do not rely on last-minute cramming sessions.
2. Thoroughly review the CBDCE *Certification for Diabetes Care and Education Specialists Handbook* so that you know exactly what to expect. Pay close attention to the content domains, subdomains, and topics. Identify your strengths, weaknesses, and knowledge gaps, so you know where to focus your studies. Review all of the supplementary resources available on the CBDCE website.
3. Create a study timeline with weekly or monthly study tasks. Be as specific as possible—identify *what* you will study, *how* you will study, and *when* you will study.
4. Use several exam prep resources that provide different benefits. For example, use a comprehensive review to build your specialty knowledge,

use this resource and other question banks to strengthen your knowledge-application and test-taking skills, and use a high-yield review to brush up on key concepts in the days leading up to the exam. Springer Publishing offers a wide range of print and online exam prep products to suit all of your study needs; visit www.springerpub.com/examprep.

5. Assess your level of knowledge and performance on practice questions and exams. Carefully consider why you may be missing certain questions. Continually analyze your strengths, weaknesses, and knowledge gaps, and adjust your study plan accordingly.

6. Minimize distraction as much as possible while you are studying. You will feel more calm, centered, and focused, which will lead to increased knowledge retention.

7. Engage in stress-reducing activities, particularly in the month leading up to the exam. Yoga, stretching, and deep-breathing exercises can be beneficial. If you are feeling frustrated or anxious while studying, take a break. Go for a walk, play with your child or pet, or finish a chore that has been weighing on you. Wait until you feel more refreshed before returning to study.

8. Focus on your health in the weeks and days before the exam. Eat balanced meals, stay hydrated, and minimize alcohol consumption. Get as much sleep as possible, particularly the night before the exam.

9. Eat a light meal before the exam but limit your liquid consumption. The clock does not stop for restroom breaks! Ensure that you know exactly where you are going and how long it will take to get there. Leave with plenty of time to spare to reduce travel-related stress and ensure that you arrive on time.

10. Remind yourself to relax and stay calm. You have prepared, and you know your stuff. Visualize the success that is just ahead of you and make it happen. When you pass, celebrate!

Pass Guarantee

If you use this resource to prepare for your exam and you do not pass, you may return it for a refund of your full purchase price. To receive a refund, you must return your product along with a copy of your original receipt and exam score report. Product must be returned and received within 180 days of the original purchase date. This excludes tax, shipping, and handling. One offer per person and address. Refunds will be issued within 8 weeks from acceptance and approval. This offer is valid for U.S. residents only. Void where prohibited. To initiate a refund, please contact customer service at CS@springerpub.com.

Part I
Practice Questions and Answers
With Rationales

Assessment of the Diabetes Continuum

1. A patient with hypertension and type 2 diabetes wants to make dietary improvements to their 2,000-kcal diet plan. A review of their food journal for the week reveals that they consumed ½ cup pinto beans. Which of the following accurately describes their legume intake compared with the recommendations outlined in the Healthy U.S. Style Eating Pattern?

   A. Sufficient; they should consume ½ cup equivalent of legumes each week
   B. Inadequate; they should consume 1 cup equivalent of legumes each week
   C. Inadequate; they should consume 1½ cup equivalents of legumes each week   *2000 KCal = 1½ Cup of beans + peas each week*
   D. Inadequate; they should consume 2 cup equivalents of legumes each week

2. A 12-year-old patient with type 2 diabetes who is being assessed for physical activity goals states that they walk their small dog for 10 minutes every day. The patient should increase their play time and physical activities to how many minutes per day?

   A. 30
   B. 45
   C. 60   *6-17 need 60 minutes of exercise per day*
   D. 90

3. What skin-related condition is most likely to be associated with diabetes?

   A. Xanthomas
   B. Eczema
   C. Cold sores
   D. Vitiligo

(See answers next page.)

1. C) Inadequate; they should consume 1½ cup equivalents of legumes each week

The Healthy U.S. Style Eating Pattern recommends that an adult following a 2,000-kcal diet consume 1½ cup equivalents of legumes (beans and peas) each week. Legumes may be considered part of the protein group, as well as the vegetable group. Legumes include kidney beans, white beans, black beans, lentils, chickpeas, pinto beans, split peas, and edamame (green soybeans). The 1½ cup recommendation is based on a total food group pattern that includes legumes as part of the vegetable subgroup and would be necessary to meet a balance of the nutrients in the recommended daily 2 cup equivalents from all of the vegetable subgroups. The ½ cup, 1 cup, and 2 cup equivalents would meet recommendations for other calorie levels but not the 2,000-kcal level.

2. C) 60

Although exercise time and intensity are difficult to track in children, the physical activity guidelines released by the U.S. Department of Health and Human Services asserts that patients ages 6 to 17 years need at least 60 minutes of physical activity per day, including aerobic, muscle-strengthening, and bone-strengthening activities. The recommendation of 60 minutes per day stems from evidence that shows a health benefit when activity reaches 500 to 1,000 metabolic equivalent (MET) minutes a week. Although 60 minutes per day is believed to be an adequate recommendation for cardio fitness and strength, evidence shows that more than 60 minutes may have additional benefits.

3. A) Xanthomas

Xanthomas are raised bumps on the skin resulting from very high levels of lipids in the blood. Skin problems like xanthomas often are associated with long-term significant elevation of glucose levels. Eczema is an itchy, scaly rash. Cold sores are red, fluid-filled blisters that form most often near the mouth and are caused by the herpes simplex virus. Vitiligo is a condition in which skin pigment is lost. Eczema, cold sores, and vitiligo are not associated with diabetes.

4. An older adult patient presents to the clinic with an A1C level of 6.3%. Which of the following is appropriate advice?

    A. "This is nothing to be concerned about because your A1C level is within the normal range."
    B. "You have evidence of uncontrolled diabetes and should be educated about initiating insulin."
    C. "You have an elevated A1C level and should start taking metformin for your diabetes."
    D. "You have an elevated A1C level that suggests prediabetes, and you should make diet and exercise changes."

5. An older adult patient with type 2 diabetes, hypertension, Stage 3 chronic kidney disease, and hepatitis C-related cirrhosis experiences morning hypoglycemia. Which of the following is the most likely reason for the hypoglycemia?

    A. Their chronic kidney disease is increasing glucose excretion
    B. They have an increased uptake of glucose from their skeletal muscles
    C. They have reduced glycogen stores due to their cirrhosis
    D. They have decreased insulin levels due to their cirrhosis

6. An adult patient assessed for diabetes is told that they have prediabetes. Which of the following fasting blood glucose (FBG) results is most likely?

    A. 53 mg/dL
    B. 87 mg/dL
    C. 115 mg/dL
    D. 136 mg/dL

fasting BG between 100-125 mg/dL is pre-diabetes

126 > diabetes range

7. A patient with complaints of excessive thirst and blurred vision presents to the ED for further evaluation. The provider suspects diabetes and orders which of the following blood tests as the most appropriate initial test to confirm the diagnosis?

    A. The A1C test, which is required for diagnostic criteria
    B. The oral glucose tolerance test (OGTT), which is the gold standard
    C. A fasting blood glucose (FBG), which is required for diagnostic confirmation
    D. A random glucose test, since the patient has already presented with symptoms

random glucose > 200mg/dL + symptoms = diabetes diagnosis

(See answers next page.)

4. D) "You have an elevated A1C level that suggests prediabetes, and you should make diet and exercise changes."
The patient should be advised of concerns because their A1C level is not within normal range. A diagnostic criterion for prediabetes is an A1C level between 5.7% and 6.4%, so this patient's A1C level is not within the normal range. The most effective intervention at this point is lifestyle therapy. Guidelines recommend considering initiating insulin when a patient's A1C is 10% or higher; therefore, initiating insulin is not advisable for this patient. Metformin could be considered, but the patient should have further testing before being told that they have diabetes.

5. C) They have reduced glycogen stores due to their cirrhosis
The skeletal muscle is the largest storage place for glycogen, but it is the liver that provides the glucose needed to raise blood glucose levels rapidly. In patients with cirrhosis of the liver, a combination of hyperinsulinemia, lack of glycogen reserves, and decreased gluconeogenic ability disrupts the process that allows rapid increases in the blood glucose level. Kidneys do have a role in glucose excretion, but chronic kidney disease is unlikely to lead to increased glucose excretion. In patients with cirrhosis, the skeletal muscle can provide amino acids for gluconeogenesis but does not contribute to increased glucose uptake. Additionally, hyperinsulinemia is a common problem; hypoinsulinemia is not.

6. C) 115 mg/dL
Prediabetes is defined as an FBG level between 100 and 125 mg/dL and can be a result of insulin resistance, impaired glucose tolerance, or both. An FBG of 53 mg/dL is clinically significant for hypoglycemia (<54 mg/dL). An FBG of 87 mg/dL is within the normal fasting glucose range of 70 to 99 mg/dL. An FBG of 136 mg/dL is in the diabetic range of 126 mg/dL or higher.

7. D) A random glucose test, since the patient has already presented with symptoms
Since the patient has already presented with symptoms, a random glucose test is the best first step. According to American Diabetes Association standards of care, a random glucose level of at least 200 mg/dL coupled with classic symptoms is sufficient for a diagnosis of diabetes. An A1C test result of at least 6.5% can support a diabetes diagnosis; however, there are imperfect correlations between A1C level and average glucose in certain individuals and populations, so it may not always be the most reliable test. An OGTT as well as an FBG are possible choices but would require repeat testing.

8. A young adult patient with type 1 diabetes is frustrated by seeing frequent high blood sugar levels before breakfast in the morning. They report that their overnight glucose levels remain above 70 and that they are not having nightmares or waking up with shakes and sweating. Which of the following is the most likely cause of the high blood sugar levels?

A. Dawn phenomenon — *does not include low BG*
B. Maturity-onset diabetes of the young
C. Somogyi effect — *rebound for when BG drops low*
D. Diabetic ketoacidosis

9. An older adult patient is taking furosemide (Lasix) for high blood pressure and wants to know about side effects. The diabetes educator explains that furosemide has potential side effects that should be monitored by blood work. Which of the following best explains the need for follow-up blood testing?

A. Furosemide can cause high sodium blood levels
B. Furosemide can cause low potassium blood levels
C. Furosemide can cause vitamin D deficiency
D. Furosemide can cause high magnesium blood levels

10. Microvascular complications of diabetes include:

A. Cerebrovascular disease
B. Coronary artery disease
C. Peripheral vascular disease
D. Nephropathy

Microvascular = retinopathy
neuropathy
nephropathy

Macrovascular — cerebrovascular
CAD.
Peripheral VD

11. Which action is an age-appropriate family concern in type 1 diabetes management during early adolescence?

A. Reassuring the child that diabetes is no one's fault — *Elementary*
B. Maintaining parental involvement in insulin and blood glucose monitoring while allowing for independent self-care during special occasions — *late elementary - middle*
C. Continuing to educate school personnel and other caregivers — *preschool elementary*
D. Monitoring for signs of depression, eating disorders, and risk-taking behaviors

(See answers next page.)

8. A) Dawn phenomenon

"Dawn phenomenon" is a term used for difficult regulation of fasting glucose in people with either type 1 or type 2 diabetes. The phenomenon is especially prevalent in people with type 1 diabetes who may not have enough circulating insulin to counteract the morning hormonal fluctuations that cause a rise in blood glucose. Maturity-onset diabetes of the young is a form of genetic defect in beta cell function. Somogyi effect is a rebound effect that occurs when glucose levels drop too low as a result of too much insulin; the body compensates with a counter-regulatory response, and the result is elevated blood sugars when evidence of hypoglycemia would be expected. The patient would have likely reported some symptoms to lead the educator to suspect hypoglycemia. Diabetic ketoacidosis is a result of insulin deficiency and is a life-threatening but reversible complication marked by severe disturbances in carbohydrate, fat, and protein metabolism.

9. B) Furosemide can cause low potassium blood levels

Furosemide can cause the body to lose potassium, an electrolyte that is needed for proper muscle and nerve function. Maintaining proper potassium replacement helps prevent this from occurring. The use of diuretics, in moderate doses, frequently combined with other medications (such as angiotensin-converting enzyme inhibitors) is a common means for preventing hypertension in people with diabetes. Furosemide can also cause low, not high, sodium (hyponatremia) and magnesium (hypomagnesemia) levels. Furosemide has no known effect on vitamin D.

10. D) Nephropathy

Microvascular complications of diabetes include nephropathy, retinopathy, and neuropathy. Macrovascular conditions include cerebrovascular, coronary artery, and peripheral vascular disease.

11. D) Monitoring for signs of depression, eating disorders, and risk-taking behaviors

Depression, eating disorders, and risk-taking behaviors are serious concerns in early adolescence that may be exacerbated by having to manage type 1 diabetes. Reassuring the child that diabetes is no one's fault should be addressed during preschool and early elementary school. Maintaining parental involvement in insulin and blood glucose monitoring while allowing for independent self-care during special occasions is important during the later elementary school years, and educating other caregivers and school personnel about diabetes is crucial during preschool and throughout elementary school.

12. A patient who was diagnosed with type 2 diabetes 2 weeks ago presents to the office for their first follow-up appointment. At that appointment, they state that they may have missed some of their medications but have made significant progress in decreasing soft drink consumption and are walking more. They also state that they are concerned about being told that their A1C level is not at the right level, and they would like to have the test repeated today. What is the best response?

    A. Inform them that lifestyle changes and knowing their A1C result are not sufficient interventions; taking their medications is more important
    B. Encourage their lifestyle changes, and obtain another A1C reading as reinforcement
    C. Encourage their lifestyle changes, and educate them that an A1C result will best reflect treatment when done at a visit 3 months in the future
    D. Encourage their lifestyle changes, and state that the A1C level is a poor indicator of glucose control; they need to check their glucose five times a day to reflect improvement

13. When counseling a patient who requires intensive therapy with frequent glucose monitoring, what is the most appropriate first intervention?

    A. Recommend continuous glucose monitoring
    B. Reassess the therapy to decrease frequency of glucose testing
    C. Screen for diabetes burnout
    D. Encourage compliance and support benefits of intensive therapy

14. A patient has type 2 diabetes. Their doctor wants them to start taking insulin, but they are hesitant and do not like the idea of needles. The patient wants to know what they can do to avoid taking insulin. What is an appropriate response in this situation?

    A. "Do you think you have done enough to control your diabetes?"
    B. "This can be stressful. Would it help you to know more about insulin?"
    C. "Maybe taking insulin is only temporary until your A1C gets better."
    D. "I understand. Needles aren't so bad. You will get used to them."

(See answers next page.)

12. C) Encourage their lifestyle changes, and educate them that an A1C result will best reflect treatment when done at a visit 3 months in the future
Lifestyle changes should be encouraged as baseline treatment for diabetes, and an A1C assessment is not recommended more frequently than every 2 to 3 months. Taking medications alone is not effective for total care management of diabetes; the patient also needs to be commended for the lifestyle changes they have made. Obtaining another A1C reading this soon after the initial one would likely not produce accurate results. The A1C is a reflection of glucose control over the past 2 to 3 months. The average life span of red blood cells (RBCs) present in the body at any given time is 2 to 3 months, and the A1C test measures the level of glycosylation of the hemoglobin. The more glucose in the blood, the more RBCs will be glycated. The higher the A1C, the poorer glucose control has been over the past 2 to 3 months. Checking glucose levels every day is encouraged, but stating that an A1C is a poor indicator of glucose control is not accurate. Additionally, requiring glucose checks five times a day is unreasonable for many patients with diabetes.

13. C) Screen for diabetes burnout
Intensive therapy can be a risk for psychological problems such as diabetes burnout, which includes feelings of frustration and hopelessness. Continuous glucose monitoring requires additional education, finances, and support, so this is not an appropriate first intervention. Decreasing the frequency of glucose testing is not beneficial because evidence shows the benefits of intensive treatment and increased monitoring. Simply encouraging compliance is not sufficient as a first intervention.

14. B) "This can be stressful. Would it help you to know more about insulin?"
Responding with "This can be stressful. Would it help you to know more about insulin?" allows for rapport and conversation, allowing the patient to express specific concerns that the diabetes educator can then address. It is unlikely that the patient's diabetes is well under control if the doctor is prescribing insulin. The diabetes educator should avoid making remarks that can provide false hope that taking insulin may be temporary. Telling the patient that they will get used to the needles is dismissive of their concerns.

15. An 82-year-old patient with dementia, heart disease, chronic kidney disease, and diabetes is being seen by a physician for a routine exam. The patient's family is concerned that the patient's blood sugar is too high and asks what ranges are considered normal for the patient. What glucose range is a reasonable target for the physician to recommend?

A. 100 to 120 mg/dL
B. 123 to 185 mg/dL
C. 147 to 217 mg/dL
D. 170 to 249 mg/dL

16. A 19-year-old patient with type 1 diabetes appears withdrawn and irritable during a clinic visit when questioned about their diabetes care. What might be an appropriate follow-up question considering their demeanor?

A. Have you lost pleasure or interest in things you used to enjoy?
B. Do you think you have enough help with your diabetes?
C. Do I need to remind you of the complications of diabetes?
D. Have you had arguments with your parents?

17. Which scenario represents contemplation as it relates to diabetes management?

A. The patient intends to start walking as exercise but is unsure when they will start   *contemplation*
B. The patient is unsure about the benefits of a diet change   *pre contemplation*
C. The patient has begun an insulin plan and has been compliant   *~action*
D. The patient intends to increase blood sugar checks to three times a day this month   *preparation*

18. A 76-year-old patient with type 2 diabetes is currently being treated with several therapies, including basal insulin. A review of their glucose checks indicates a range from 75 to 185 mg/dL. What glucose level is recommended to be a lower-end target range?

A. 65 mg/dL   *Older Adults do not want*
B. 70 mg/dL   *a glucose < 80 mg/dL*
C. 75 mg/dL
D. 80 mg/dL

(See answers next page.)

15. C) 147 to 217 mg/dL
A blood glucose range of 147 to 217 mg/dL is recommended because it corre-lates to a less stringent A1C goal of less than 8%. A less stringent A1C goal helps prevent dehydration, symptoms of hyperglycemia or hypoglycemia, and weight loss, and it facilitates wound healing. The other ranges are either too low or too high to meet this patient's specific needs.

16. B) Do you think you have enough help with your diabetes?
Because the patient seems irritated when questioned about their diabetes care, delving further into their diabetes management may help the educator assess for diabetes burnout before moving on to assess for other issues. Asking about the loss of pleasure or interest would be more beneficial when screening for depres-sion. Scare tactics about complications are not recommended. Asking about argu-ments would be appropriate if assessing for family conflicts, but this is not the initial goal for this patient.

17. A) The patient intends to start walking as exercise but is unsure when they will start
Contemplation is demonstrated by intent and thinking of a plan that does not begin in the immediate future. Being unsure about establishing a goal at all, like diet change, is an example of precontemplation. Already beginning a plan repre-sents action. Having the intention to change within the foreseeable future illus-trates preparation.

18. D) 80 mg/dL
In older adults, hypoglycemia, or serum glucose levels lower than 80 mg/dL, can result in poor outcomes, including traumatic falls and exacerbation of comorbid conditions.

19. Which symptom would be the mostly likely sign of neuroglycopenic hypoglycemia in a person with diabetes?

    A. Confusion — *neuroglycopenic (mental + behavioral).*
    B. Tremors
    C. Sweating   } *Adrenergic*
    D. Palpitations

20. A patient states that they have been collecting healthy recipes and have recently purchased several exercise videos. Which stage of change is this patient demonstrating?

    A. Precontemplation
    B. Contemplation
    C. Preparation
    D. Action

21. A diabetes educator sees an adult patient with type 2 diabetes for a routine follow-up visit. The patient is upset and states that they have just been diagnosed with retinopathy and fear losing their sight. What is an appropriate intervention?

    A. Screen for diabetes burnout
    B. Screen for depression
    C. Screen for diabetes distress — *reacting to factors associated w/progression of diabetes*
    D. Screen for anxiety

22. Which factor is being assessed with the question, "Since you test your blood sugar four times a day, how many glucose test strips do you need to take with you on a 2-week vacation?"

    A. Diabetes literacy = *reading skills*
    B. Diabetes numeracy = *math skills*
    C. General health beliefs
    D. Concrete thinking skills

(See answers next page.)

19. A) Confusion

Neuroglycopenic hypoglycemia symptoms include mental and behavioral symptoms such as lethargy, dizziness, and confusion. Adrenergic (also neurogenic or sympathoadrenal) symptoms of hypoglycemia include tremors, sweating, and palpitations.

20. C) Preparation

This patient is preparing to make some changes to their lifestyle in the near future. People in this stage of change are likely to experiment with small changes such as collecting recipes and buying exercise videos. In the precontemplation stage, change is not considered at all. In the contemplation stage of change, the patient is ambivalent about changing and begins to assess the barriers and benefits of changes. In the action stage, a patient is already actively working to change something about themself or their lifestyle.

21. C) Screen for diabetes distress

Diabetes distress can be experienced when a patient is reacting to factors associated with the progression and course of diabetes. The Diabetes Distress Scale is a way to specifically screen for diabetes distress. Diabetes burnout occurs when a person is feeling frustrated and like a failure in managing their diabetes. Depression and anxiety are often common among individuals dealing with diabetes, but these mood disorders are more generalized with a wider range of symptoms and may not be related directly to the diabetes.

22. B) Diabetes numeracy

Limited diabetes numeracy may be an important factor affecting diabetes care and treatment. Research has demonstrated that lower numeracy skills can impact efficacy, self-care behaviors, and overall glycemic outcomes. Literacy is important when assessing reading skills, such as medication labels or travel tip instructions. Health beliefs are relevant in the assessment of a patient's perception of the disease and treatment. Concrete thinking would apply if the educator was asking about the logic and general concept of glucose monitoring.

23. An adult patient with type 1 diabetes comes to the office for a routine follow-up visit. Glucose records show an average of 70 to 80 mg/dL after lunch and dinner. Fasting and premeal results show an average of 110 to 140 mg/dL. The patient uses an insulin pump. Which change to the pump setting is recommended?

    A. Reduce the basal rate
    B. Decrease the insulin-to-carbohydrate ratio rate for lunch and dinner
    C. Modify the correction factor to give less insulin
    D. Increase the insulin-to-carbohydrate ratio rate for lunch and dinner

24. An 18-year-old patient with type 1 diabetes wants to understand why their A1C has increased to 10.0. The patient's parents are present and state that they are also worried about the patient's glucose control and have begun to ask more frequently about what the patient is eating and how much insulin the patient takes. What is the most appropriate intervention?

    A. Suggest ways to reduce risk of miscarried helping
    B. Praise the parents for supportive interventions
    C. Encourage the parents to let their child be independent
    D. Assess for concerns or signs of diabetes burnout

25. Continuous glucose monitoring is most appropriate for a pediatric patient who:

    A. Has never experienced a severe hypoglycemic episode
    B. Has hypoglycemic unawareness
    C. Does not have nocturnal hypoglycemia
    D. Has demonstrated good glycemic control for at least 1 year

26. A 29-year-old patient, newly diagnosed with diabetes, is being seen for home discharge education. The patient asks whether they can still eat pizza and have an occasional beer. What would be a priority goal for the diabetes educator at this session?

    A. Understanding the relationship among food, insulin, and blood glucose
    B. Encouraging protein intake of 10% to 20% of calories to support health
    C. Recommending specific carbohydrates and carbohydrate requirements
    D. Discussing alcohol's effects on diabetes

(See answers next page.)

23. B) Decrease the insulin-to-carbohydrate ratio rate for lunch and dinner

Decreasing the insulin-to-carbohydrate ratio corrects post-meal glucose. Decreasing the basal rate would impact fasting glucose. Correction factor modifications would correct pre-meal glucose. Increasing the insulin-to-carbohydarate ratio would be necessary to correct hyperglycemia.

24. A) Suggest ways to reduce risk of miscarried helping

Miscarried helping is the term used when the support attempts by family members or friends are excessive, untimely, or inappropriate. Improving communication about support and boundaries in care often helps avoid failed attempts to help the patient. Parental oversight can be supportive but not always effective in supporting an adolescent's transition to competent self-care. Additionally, transfer of responsibility should occur gradually, and the patient should not be totally independent. With diabetes burnout, the patient shows signs of frustration and hopelessness.

25. B) Has hypoglycemic unawareness

Continuous glucose monitoring is most appropriate for a child who has hypoglycemic unawareness. Continuous glucose monitoring may also be appropriate for the child who requires frequent blood glucose monitoring, has severe hypoglycemic episodes, has nocturnal hypoglycemia, has broad variations in glucose levels (regardless of A1C), has suboptimal glycemic control with A1C exceeding the target range, and/or has A1C levels less than 7% and wishes to maintain target glycemic control while limiting hypoglycemia risk.

26. A) Understanding the relationship among food, insulin, and blood glucose

Understanding the relationship among food, insulin, and blood glucose to improve blood glucose control is the patient's most immediate need and the educator's priority goal. Further topics beyond these essentials can be approached as the patient demonstrates proficiency and readiness to learn more specific and advanced topics, such as specific questions regarding different food groups and alcohol.

27. Which religious observance should the diabetes educator discuss with patients regarding the risks of hypoglycemia, glucose monitoring, and medication timing?

    A. Ramadan
    B. Passover
    C. Rosh Hashanah
    D. Purim

28. Which condition is a symptom of diabetes?

    A. Hyperactive behavior
    B. Weight gain
    C. Loss of appetite
    D. Polyuria

29. A patient with type 2 diabetes, high blood pressure, high cholesterol, and a long history of tobacco use presents to the doctor's office. Labs show an estimated glomerular filtration rate (eGFR) of 39 mL/min/1.73 m². Which assessment best describes the patient's kidney function?

    A. Stage 2 kidney damage with mildly decreased eGFR
    B. Stage 3 kidney damage with moderately decreased eGFR
    C. Stage 4 kidney damage with severely decreased eGFR
    D. Stage 5 kidney failure

30. A patient with type 2 diabetes, high blood pressure, and high cholesterol weighs 249 lb and is 69 inches tall. The patient is being seen by a diabetes educator. They discuss nutrition, and the patient reports that their meal from the night before was a bowl of canned vegetable soup, a deli turkey sandwich with reduced-fat cheese, some snack pickles, and an unsweetened iced tea. Based on the patient's recall, which of their medical conditions requires dietary changes?

    A. Diabetes
    B. High cholesterol
    C. High blood pressure
    D. Obesity

(*See answers next page.*)

27. A) Ramadan

Ramadan is a Muslim holiday that entails fasting from sunrise to sunset. The delay before eating and the inconsistent meal patterns present a risk for hypoglycemia, especially in insulin-dependent patients and patients with a history of hypoglycemia unawareness. A plan of care would be to assess the patient's decision to fast and have a further assessment and instruction plan during observation of Ramadan. Passover, Rosh Hashanah, and Purim are all Jewish holidays that include feasting and alcohol. The education topics would not include risks of fasting but would include the risk of alcohol-induced hypoglycemia.

28. D) Polyuria

Symptoms of diabetes include polyuria, polydipsia, fatigue, polyphagia, weight loss, and blurred vision. Hyperactivity, weight gain, and anorexia are not common symptoms of diabetes.

29. B) Stage 3 kidney damage with moderately decreased eGFR

Stage 3 kidney damage with moderately decreased eGFR includes an eGFR range of 30 to 59 mL/min/1.73 m². The eGFR range in Stage 2 kidney damage is 60 to 89 mL/min/1.73 m². In Stage 4 kidney disease, the eGFR range is 15 to 29 mL/min/1.73 m². In Stage 5 kidney failure, the eGFR is less than 15 mL/min/1.73 m².

30. C) High blood pressure

The meal includes three high-sodium items: canned soup, deli turkey, and pickles. Evidence supports a sodium-reduced diet to help manage high blood pressure. The patient's choices are not high enough in fat, carbohydrates, sugars, or calories to warrant changing the diet to manage cholesterol, diabetes, or obesity.

31. A patient's insulin pen self-administration is being assessed. The patient cleans and attaches a 4-mm pen needle, dials the dose, inserts the needle into the skin, fully depresses the button, withdraws after 10 seconds, properly detaches and disposes of the needle, and replaces the pen cap. Which corrective teaching is needed?

    A. The need to clean the skin with alcohol
    B. Pinching the skin before injection
    C. Leaving the needle in too long after infection
    D. The need to prime the needle before injection

32. Glyburide is a commonly prescribed antidiabetic medication because of its cost-effectiveness. Which potential side effect of glyburide is of the greatest patient concern?

    A. Hypoglycemia   + weight gain
    B. Weight loss
    C. Gastrointestinal side effects
    D. Edema

    Brand Names
    Diabeta
    Glycron
    Glynase Pres-Tab
    Micronase

33. An older adult patient with a history of type 2 diabetes presents to the ED complaining of foot pain and swelling. Upon examination, the right foot is warm to the touch and appears red. What would be a possible concern?

    A. Hammer toe — bone deformity
    B. Charcot foot — warmth, redness, pain, swelling
    C. Early foot ulcer — callus, irritation, wound
    D. Peripheral artery disease — leg fatigue, ↓ pedal pulses

34. A 26-year-old patient with gestational diabetes is meeting with a diabetes educator. Which monitoring and self-care recommendation would be appropriate for this patient?

    A. Check A1C every 6 to 8 weeks
    B. Limit exercise due to hypoglycemia risk
    C. Eat additional carbohydrates with each meal
    D. Self-monitor blood glucose up to 5 to 7 times per day

    ↳ euglycemia is goal for pt
       ↳ good / normal range BG

(See answers next page.)

31. D) The need to prime the needle before injection
Insulin pens require priming before injection. It is not absolutely necessary to clean the skin with alcohol before an injection. Needles smaller than 8 mm are small enough that pinching the skin for an injection is not required. It is generally necessary to ensure complete injection by waiting 10 seconds after the injection.

32. A) Hypoglycemia
Glyburide, although inexpensive, carries the risk of hypoglycemia. An additional risk is weight gain, not weight loss. Gastrointestinal side effects are often associated with metformin, not glyburide. Edema is a risk with thiazolidinediones, not sulfonylureas.

33. B) Charcot foot
Charcot foot presents with warmth, pain, swelling, and redness and is a risk associated with type 2 diabetes. Hammer toe is a bony deformity that can cause discomfort but would present as more of a joint abnormality. An early foot ulcer may present as a callus or irritation. Peripheral artery disease would present with leg fatigue and decreased pedal pulses.

34. D) Self-monitor blood glucose up to 5 to 7 times per day
The diabetes educator should recommend that this patient monitor their blood glucose 5 to 7 times each day; euglycemia is a primary goal for patient and fetal safety. An A1C test every 4 to 6 weeks is recommended. Physical activity is included as lifestyle management of gestational diabetes and has been shown to have more benefits than risks. Carbohydrate restriction to within assessed calorie needs demonstrates improved outcomes.

35. What is a common first-line medication expected to be prescribed for a patient with history of high cholesterol?

    A. Fenofibrate *— fibrate — ↑ triglycerides*
    B. Atorvastatin
    C. Gemfibrozil *— fibrate — ↑ triglycerides*
    D. Ezetimibe

36. Obstructive sleep apnea (OSA) can be a common comorbidity with diabetes. Which is a risk factor for OSA?

    A. Smoking *— Risk! 3 x as high*
    B. High blood pressure
    C. Chronic cough
    D. Snoring *— symptom of OSA*

37. An adult patient with a 7-year history of type 2 diabetes comes to the office for a routine follow-up visit. The patient reports that they are not yet able to increase physical activity to 150 minutes a week; have reduced some carbo-hydrates, such as rice and pasta; and are checking glucose at least twice a day as recommended. Blood pressure is 145/92 mmHg, A1C is 7.2%, low-density lipoprotein cholesterol is 95, high-density lipoprotein is 37, and triglycerides are 142. The patient's records show an annual foot exam, an eye exam 2 years ago, and a urine test 6 months ago. Which "ABC" goals are not being met?

    A. A1C and blood pressure
    B. A1C and cholesterol
    C. Blood pressure and cholesterol
    D. A1C only

    ABCs =
    A1C
    Blood pressure
    cholesterol
    Goals = < 140/90 BP
    LDP < 100
    HDL   A1C < 7%

38. What is the recommended age for diabetes testing regardless of individual risk?

    A. 35
    B. 40
    C. 45
    D. 50

35. B) Atorvastatin
Atorvastatin is a recommended as an initial dyslipidemia treatment. Fenofibrate and gemfibrozil are not statins but fibrates, and would therefore be considered if triglyceride levels are higher than 1,000 mg/dL. However, these are not first-line treatments. Additionally, gemfibrozil is not typically combined with a statin because of concerns for rhabdomyolysis. Ezetimibe is a second-line treatment and is not a statin but a selective cholesterol absorption inhibitor.

36. A) Smoking
Smoking is a risk factor for OSA; smokers are three times more likely to have OSA than their nonsmoking counterparts. High blood pressure is a common clinical finding with OSA but not a risk factor. Nasal congestion and allergies can be a risk factor, but not chronic cough. Snoring is a symptom of OSA, not a risk factor.

37. A) A1C and blood pressure
The "ABCs" of diabetes refer to goals for A1C, blood pressure, and cholesterol. The goals include a blood pressure goal of less than 140/90 mm Hg, low-density lipoprotein goal less than 100 mg/dL, and A1C goal of less than 7%. This patient does not meet his goals for A1C or blood pressure. His cholesterol is within the goal limits.

38. C) 45
For all people, testing is recommended beginning at age 45. Testing should be done at a younger age if risk factors exist. Because the risk of diabetes increases with age, the consensus is to test by age 45 rather than wait until age 50.

39. A patient's glucose record shows ranges of 165 to 276 mg/dL. The patient's A1C for the current visit is 7.5%. Which statement could explain the discrepancy?

    A. The patient has iron deficiency anemia
    B. The patient has chronic alcohol intake
    C. The patient has untreated hypertriglyceridemia
    D. The patient has had a recent surgery

40. An inpatient diabetes educator is assessing and educating a patient newly diagnosed with type 2 diabetes. Part of the provider's responsibility is to explain how to select and use a glucose meter. Which finding is most likely to affect the information provided about meter selection?

    A. The patient correctly demonstrates strip insertion
    B. The patient has a history of hepatitis C
    C. The patient has a tremor
    D. The patient works outside in a warm environment

41. A 10-year-old patient with type 1 diabetes presents with abdominal pain, vomiting, dehydration, and loss of consciousness. What is the most likely cause?

    A. Ketosis or ketoacidosis
    B. Glomerulosclerosis
    C. Diabetic cystopathy
    D. Cerebrovascular disease

42. When 80% to 90% of the beta-cell mass has been destroyed and the individual's insulin secretory capacity becomes insufficient to normally regulate hepatic glucose production, what can the diabetes educator expect to see first?

    A. Postprandial hyperglycemia
    B. Progressive fasting hyperglycemia
    C. Glucose toxicity
    D. Glucosuria

(*See answers next page.*)

39. D) The patient has had a recent surgery

Most likely, the patient has had a recent surgery. Acute blood loss from events such as a surgery can be associated with a falsely low A1C. Iron deficiency anemia, chronic alcohol intake, and hypertriglyceridemia can cause falsely elevated A1C.

40. C) The patient has a tremor

A tremor suggests dexterity impairment, which requires a meter and strip that has an adequate size and shape for ease of use. Strip insertion is a component of monitoring technique. A history of hepatitis C would be important for meter safety education rather than meter choice. The fact that the patient works outside in a warm environment would be more important for education on potential sources of error.

41. A) Ketosis or ketoacidosis

Abdominal pain, vomiting, dehydration, and loss of consciousness are all signs and symptoms of ketosis or ketoacidosis, often missed in the child or infant who is significantly ill. Glomerulosclerosis is a class of renal histopathological changes that characterize diabetic nephropathy. Diabetic cystopathy is the diminished sensation of bladder fullness and is an autonomic syndrome associated with diabetes. Cerebrovascular disease includes intermittent dizziness, transient loss of vision, slurring of speech, and paresthesia, or weakness of one arm or leg. These conditions do not align with the patient's specific signs and symptoms the way ketosis and and ketoacidosis do.

42. A) Postprandial hyperglycemia

Postprandial hyperglycemia (along with some decrease in peripheral glucose utilization) is the first and only sign of a failure to adequately suppress hepatic glucose production during mealtime absorption. As insulin secretion is further compromised, progressive fasting hyperglycemia occurs. Hyperglycemia sometimes further compromises glucose utilization by reducing the number and/or activity of glucose transporters available on both insulin-dependent and non-insulin-dependent tissues; this occurs later and is known as glucose toxicity. Glucosuria occurs when plasma glucose concentration exceeds the renal threshold of about 180 mg/dL and is not seen before postprandial hyperglycemia.

43. A 27-year-old patient is diagnosed with gestational diabetes. The food record shows two slices of bread, yogurt, and berries at breakfast; 1 cup rice with stir-fry at lunch; ½ potato, ½ cup peas, fish, and pudding at dinner. In addition to the meals, the patient has three snacks a day that may include fruit or a few crackers with cheese or peanut butter. What is the best recommendation for the patient's eating choices?

    A. Decrease the amount of snacks
    B. Add a carbohydrate to lunch
    C. Decrease carbohydrate at breakfast
    D. Add a carbohydrate to dinner

44. A patient with type 2 diabetes has been struggling with making proper dietary changes and expresses frustration that their job as a truck driver limits them from being able to make the changes they know they should make. Which response by the diabetes educator is the most appropriate?

    A. "Do you feel overwhelmed by your diabetes?"
    B. "Are you letting your job be an excuse for not making changes to your diet?"
    C. "How could a reward help you to be successful?"
    D. "How can you see yourself overcoming that barrier?"

45. What is the primary benefit of fructosamine testing?

    A. It is more accurate than A1C
    B. It can be checked weekly instead of checking blood glucose daily
    C. It can detect overall changes in blood glucose control over a shorter time span than A1C
    D. It can help determine whether someone has type 1 or type 2 diabetes

46. A patient with type 2 diabetes provides an activity history. The patient states that although they have a desk job, they try to stretch and get up every hour. The patient walks 45 minutes 4 days a week and lifts weights twice a week. What can be assessed about the patient's activity needs?

    A. The patient is sedentary at work and should get up every 30 minutes
    B. The patient is not walking enough and should walk 30 minutes every day
    C. The patient is not getting enough resistance exercise and should add a day
    D. The patient is meeting activity goals and should aim to maintain the goals

(See answers next page.)

43. C) Decrease carbohydrate at breakfast

This patient should decrease carbohydrate intake at breakfast. It is common for glucose levels to be elevated in the morning. Limiting breakfast carbohydrate may benefit morning glucose control. Three snacks a day are recommended as part of a consistent meal plan for gestational diabetes. The lunch and dinner meals are both between 45 and 60 g of carbohydrate, which is appropriate.

44. D) "How can you see yourself overcoming that barrier?"

Asking the patient how they can see themselves overcoming that barrier presents an appropriate problem-focused intervention that can lead to the patient formulating strategies to achieve the desired goal. Asking if the patient feels overwhelmed is an emotional intervention-focused question and likely not helpful in this scenario. Asking the patient about the job being an excuse is not supportive or therapeutic. Asking about a reward would not be supportive unless there is additional resistance to change that would require a contract for change/problem-focused intervention.

45. C) It can detect overall changes in blood glucose control over a shorter time span than A1C

Fructosamine testing can detect overall changes in blood glucose control over a shorter time span than the A1C. Fructosamine levels indicate the level of blood glucose control over the past 2 or 3 weeks. The test can be clinically beneficial, such as when evaluating a treatment change or assessing glucose control in a patient with a condition that would affect the A1C. As with many other tests, fructosamine testing can be inaccurate in certain settings, such as with renal and liver disease. It is not intended to be a routinely used test to replace daily monitoring, nor does the test translate well into average glucose levels, making it a limiting diagnostic test.

46. A) The patient is sedentary at work and should get up every 30 minutes

The patient is sedentary at work and needs to get up every 30 minutes. Current activity guidelines support interrupting sedentary behavior every 30 minutes. This patient is not breaking up sedentary behavior sufficiently, although they are meeting the 150 minutes of planned activity and 2 or more days of resistance exercise. Overall, however, this patient is not meeting activity goals according to recommendations.

47. A 76-year-old patient with a history of congestive heart failure has recurring hospitalizations for exacerbation of congestive heart failure. A diabetes educator is visiting the patient and reviews home medications. Which medication is of concern specific to the congestive heart failure and should be brought to the physician's attention?

    A. Glyburide — hypoglycemia
    B. Pioglitazone — thiazolidinedione = ↑ risk for edema + heart disease
    C. Acarbose — GI side effects
    D. Metformin — GI side effects

48. An adult patient with type 2 diabetes is admitted for infection and hypoglycemia. The A1C is 10.4, but the patient does not understand what that means in terms of health. The patient says they do not use their meter because it "doesn't work" for them. The patient understands the seriousness of diabetes because their father, who had diabetes, lost a leg and was on dialysis. Which learning goals should be reviewed first with this patient?

    A. Skills of blood glucose monitoring
    B. Goals to lower A1C
    C. Seriousness of complications
    D. Medication compliance

49. Increased waist circumference is a major criterion for the clinical diagnosis of metabolic syndrome. Which are the cutoffs for increased risk?

    A. 35 inches for women and 40 inches for men
    B. 40 inches for women and 45 inches for men   735 W
    C. 45 inches for women and 50 inches for men   740 M
    D. 35 inches for both women and men

50. Which of the following is a simple tool to assess a patient's readiness to change?

    A. The Newest Vital Sign — Health Hx
    B. Ruler method — gauges readiness to change + confidence in behavior change
    C. Patient Health Questionnaire-2
    D. Berlin Questionnaire — sleep apnea exam

(See answers next page.)

47. B) Pioglitazone

Pioglitazone is a thiazolidinedione, which has an increased risk for edema and heart failure. Glyburide's key side effect is hypoglycemia, the most common complication with acarbose is gastrointestinal side effects, and metformin has gastrointestinal effects and is contraindicated with reduced renal function; these three drugs are not contraindicated in the presence of congestive heart failure.

48. A) Skills of blood glucose monitoring

It is important to review this patient's blood glucose monitoring skills first. Learning how to monitor blood glucose is a first step toward managing A1C and reducing complications. Furthermore, reviewing complications first may be interpreted as noncollaborative, and using threats for compliance is not effective for successful behavior changes. There is not enough information to assume lack of engagement with medication compliance.

49. A) 35 inches for women and 40 inches for men

A waist circumference of greater than 35 inches for women and greater than 40 inches for men is considered the criterion for metabolic syndrome. Many clinicians believe that clinical diagnosis of visceral adiposity may be more important than body mass index, body weight, or even percentage of total body fat. Waist circumferences of 40 or 45 inches for women and 45 or 50 inches for men are above the cutoffs for increased risk, and 35 inches is below the cutoff for men.

50. B) Ruler method

The Ruler method is a tool used to gauge a patient's readiness to change and confidence in behavior change. For example, "On a scale of 0 to 10, how important is it for you to change your diet?" The Newest Vital Sign assesses health literacy. The Patient Health Questionnaire-2 assesses for depression. The Berlin Questionnaire assesses for sleep apnea.

51. An A1C of 9.5% represents an estimated average glucose (eAG) of:

A. 169 mg/dL
B. 226 mg/dL
C. 298 mg/dL
D. 375 mg/dL

[handwritten: $28.7 \times 9.5 - 46.7 = $ eag of 226]

52. A patient with a 12-year history of type 1 diabetes complains of increased burning and tingling in the extremities. An assessment finds no sensation to a monofilament test, no ankle reflexes, and no vibration sensation. What is the most likely diagnosis?

A. Autonomic neuropathy
B. Peripheral arterial disease
C. Sciatica
D. Peripheral neuropathy

53. Upon examination of a patient's injection sites, hard nodules can be felt. What is a plausible cause?

A. The patient is reusing needles
B. The patient is pulling the needle out too quickly
C. The patient is not rotating injection sites
D. The patient is injecting the needle too deeply

54. An 18-year-old patient with type 1 diabetes has an established insulin pump for diabetes management. The patient has just joined a cross-country running team and is concerned about becoming hypoglycemic after every training session. The patient consumes a 15-g portion of glucose tablets about every 15 minutes. Which statement explains this patient's condition?

A. The patient is not consuming enough glucose tablets
B. The patient is not lowering the basal rate of the insulin pump
C. The patient should be tested for autonomic neuropathy
D. The patient needs a continual glucose monitor

55. A 79-year-old patient needs home supplies for glucose monitoring. What physical feature of the blood glucose meter is the most appropriate first consideration in helping this patient choose which product to purchase?

A. Required blood sample size
B. Size of the blood glucose meter
C. Memory capacity
D. Speech-output capability

(See answers next page.)

51. B) 226 mg/dL
An A1C of 9.5% represents an eAG of 226 mg/dL. The formula for calculating eAG from A1C is 28.7 x A1C – 46.7 = eAG. This eAG result does not necessarily mean that the blood glucose has been stable at 226 over the past few months; the blood glucose could have ranged from 40 to 300 mg/dL. The use of eAG has not been widely accepted by clinicians. The levels 169, 298, and 375 mg/dL are incorrect results when calculating for eAG.

52. D) Peripheral neuropathy
Loss of protective sensation indicates the presence of peripheral neuropathy and is a common risk concern for patients with diabetes that requires screenings. Autonomic neuropathy presents with hypoglycemia unawareness, resting tachycardia, and gastroparesis. Peripheral artery disease has clinical indicators of decreased walking speed and decreased pedal pulses. Sciatica manifests with pain symptoms that start in the upper extremities and progress down to the lower extremities.

53. C) The patient is not rotating injection sites
The patient is not rotating injection sites. Rotating sites is a recommended way to prevent lipohypertrophy, which manifests in hard nodules. Reusing needles is not recommended for safety and hygiene. Burning or redness may occur when insulin comes into contact with the skin from pulling the needle out too quickly. Injecting the needle too deeply when using a longer needle could make the injection intramuscular, but it is not associated with lipohypertrophy.

54. B) The patient is not lowering the basal rate of the insulin pump
Reducing the basal rate is appropriate to account for intense physical activity. The patient is correctly consuming the recommended 15 g of glucose tablets (carbohydrate) every 15 minutes, per guidelines. Autonomic neuropathy would be a concern if the patient demonstrated lack of awareness of hypoglycemia. A continual glucose monitor could provide improved feedback on glucose; however, only having improved monitoring would not prevent or explain the recurring hypoglycemia.

55. B) Size of the blood glucose meter
Considering the size of the meter takes dexterity into consideration. Dexterity is the most likely issue for an older adult patient and is therefore the most appropriate first consideration. Blood sample size and memory capacity are recommended considerations for children. Speech-output capacity is beneficial for a patient with visual impairment, not necessarily for an older adult patient.

56. Which insulin preparation should be taken at every mealtime?

A. Glargine — No long action

B. Lispro — RAPID Before meals

C. Neutral protamine hagedorn (NPH) — Twice a day — intermediate acting

D. Detemir — No-long acting

57. A 75-year-old patient with type 2 diabetes, congestive heart failure, chronic kidney disease, and hypertension has been discharged from the hospital with orders for home health wound care. The patient says that their doctor said the patient's A1C was too high. Which is an appropriate A1C goal for this patient?

A. No goal given his health complications and life expectancy

B. A less stringent goal of 7% to 8%

C. A more stringent goal of 6% to 7%

D. A standard goal of 7%

58. Which self-care behavior is most appropriate to assess when giving discharge instructions to a patient newly diagnosed with diabetes?

A. Carbohydrate counting — Advanced

B. Insulin adjustment — Advanced

C. Monitoring — BASIC — new diabetic

D. Foot care technique — Advanced

59. Which generation most likely expects a PowerPoint lecture approach in the classroom? 1965-80

A. Generation X

B. Baby boomers

C. Millennials — 1981-1995

D. Generation Z — 1996-2010

60. A 52-year-old patient with type 2 diabetes was recently admitted to the hospital for a stroke. The patient is referred to diabetes education for uncontrolled diabetes. What should be the area of focus for this patient?

A. Educate on treatment goals

B. Review self-management skills

C. Identify barriers to self-management

D. Discuss resources for education

(See answers next page.)

56. B) Lispro
Lispro is a rapid-acting analog insulin and an optimal insulin to manage mealtime glucose control. Glargine and detemir are both long-acting basal analog insulins that work best as a daily dose. NPH is an intermediate-acting insulin and is preferred for cost reasons but has a longer action and works best as a twice-a-day insulin.

57. B) A less stringent goal of 7% to 8%
Multiple factors should be used in managing hyperglycemia. They include risks associated with hypoglycemia, disease duration, life expectancy, relevant comorbidities, established vascular complications, attitude, and resources and support. In this case, a goal should be established, but in consideration of complications and life expectancy, a goal of more than 7% would be most realistic for this patient.

58. C) Monitoring
Discharge planning should cover some basic areas of knowledge, which include monitoring. Carbohydrate counting, insulin adjustment, and foot care technique are advanced knowledge areas that would not be appropriate at this stage and are more appropriate for outpatient follow-up.

59. A) Generation X
Generation X (people born between 1965 and 1980) expect PowerPoint lecture slides featuring graphs and bullet point presentations. Baby boomers (1946–1964) expect a more interactive and visual tool learning style. Millennials (1981–1995) appreciate group work and technology. Generation Z (1996–2010) expect learning to incorporate distance and social network learning.

60. C) Identify barriers to self-management
The patient has experienced new complicating factors. It would be appropriate to identify any factors that are affecting the patient's self-management and behavioral goals. Educating on treatment goals and discussing resources for education are more appropriate to focus on at diagnosis. Review of self-management skills should occur at a regular annual assessment.

61. A patient who presents to the ED is found to have ketoacidosis without significant hyperglycemia, a condition known as euglycemic diabetic ketoacidosis.
What medication is the likely cause of the patient's condition?

   A. Sodium-glucose cotransporter 2 (SGLT2) inhibitor
   B. Glucagon-like peptide 1 receptor (GLP-1) agonist — GI / pancreatitis / thyroid tumors
   C. Dipeptidyl peptidase 4 (DPP-4) inhibitor — HF
   D. Sulfonylurea — hypoglycemia + weight gain

62. A patient who has type 1 diabetes comes to the physician's office with ketone
production and hyperglycemia. What is the most likely cause?

   A. Significant insulin deficiency
   B. Recent childbirth
   C. Rapid weight gain
   D. Very little recent physical activity

63. Type 1 diabetes is now considered to have three distinct stages. Which stage
is symptomatic?

   A. Stage 1   > antibody > stage
   B. Stage 2
   C. Stage 3
   D. All stages

64. Which food is a high source of alpha-linolenic acid?

   A. Fatty fish — EPA/DHA
   B. Olive oil — monosaturated fat
   C. Butter — saturated fat
   D. Flax seed — ALA

65. A patient with type 2 diabetes has a history of high blood pressure and presents with a repeat blood pressure of 148/96 mmHg. The patient reports fair
compliance with lifestyle changes and has stopped smoking. They are not
currently on any blood pressure therapy. What would be an appropriate next
treatment?

   A. Angiotensin-converting enzyme (ACE) inhibitor
   B. Diuretic
   C. Calcium channel blocker   > second tier approach
   D. Beta-blocker

(See answers next page.)

61. A) Sodium-glucose cotransporter 2 (SGLT2) inhibitor

Research and reports have led the U.S. Food and Drug Administration (FDA) to issue warnings about the risk of ketoacidosis with the use of SGLT2 inhibitors. GLP-1 receptor agonists often have gastrointestinal adverse effects and a disadvantage in animal testing showing increased incidence of C-cell hyperplasia and medullary thyroid tumors. DPP-4 inhibitors have a guideline risk of increased hospitalizations for heart failure. Sulfonylureas carry a risk of hypoglycemia and weight gain.

62. A) Significant insulin deficiency

Significant insulin deficiency results in rising glucose levels and allows fat metabolism to occur. Ketone production is also likely to occur when someone has extreme or rapid weight loss, not gain; during pregnancy if there are insufficient calories to meet increased energy needs; or with extreme exercise.

63. C) Stage 3

Current research has established three stages of type 1 diabetes. Stage 3 is the highest stage and is associated with established clinical symptoms of hyperglycemia. Stages 1 and 2 are antibody-established stages of type 1 diabetes, but these stages are presymptomatic.

64. D) Flax seed

Flax seed is an established beneficial source of alpha-linolenic acid for prevention and treatment of cardiovascular disease. Fatty fish is a high source of eicosapentaenoic acid (EPA) and docosahexaenoic acid (DHA), and olive oil is a good source of monounsaturated fats, which are also supportive of cardiovascular health. Butter is high in saturated fat, which is contraindicated for cardiovascular health.

65. A) Angiotensin-converting enzyme (ACE) inhibitor

American Diabetes Association standards of care state that an ACE inhibitor or angiotensin receptor blocker at the maximum dose for therapy is the recommended first-line treatment for hypertension. Diuretics, calcium channel blockers, and beta-blockers can all provide additional benefits but are considered second-tier and are taken in combination with other hypertension therapies.

66. An adult patient has type 2 diabetes, hypertension, and chronic kidney disease. The patient eats three meals a day. A 24-hour dietary recall reveals this information:
    - Breakfast: 1 biscuit, 1 egg, and ½ cup orange juice
    - Lunch: 1 chicken stir-fry frozen meal
    - Dinner: ½ cup packaged yellow rice, 1 small corn muffin, 1 piece of white fish, and 1 cup broccoli

    What dietary education does this patient need?

    A. Reducing dietary sodium
    B. Healthy fat choices
    C. Carbohydrate counting
    D. Snack planning

67. A 15-year-old patient with type 1 diabetes is struggling to consistently monitor their glucose. They state that for 3 months they have been using the agreed-upon plan to use a smartphone app to remind them to check their glucose levels. Which action is an appropriate evaluation of this plan?

    A. Addressing how to properly check and log their glucose levels
    B. Asking what the patient wants to gain from improved monitoring
    C. Comparing the patient's previous logs to their current log
    D. Recording the patient's log records in the patient chart

68. A patient with type 2 diabetes is admitted for treatment of an acute infection. Admission glucose is 275 and A1C is 7.4%. What can be inferred from these values?

    A. The patient's diabetes is uncontrolled
    B. The patient has recently experienced stress
    C. The patient is maintaining good glucose control
    D. The patient has recently started a new medication

(See answers next page.)

66. A) Reducing dietary sodium

The patient needs education in how to reduce dietary sodium. The dietary recall reveals many established high-sodium foods——biscuits, frozen meals, and processed foods such as packaged yellow rice. The history of hypertension and chronic kidney disease would support recommendations for sodium restriction in the diet. Overall, the dietary recall does not provide much evidence for unhealthy fat choices or inconsistent carbohydrate intake. Snack planning is not greatly indicated because the patient demonstrates a consistent meal plan.

67. C) Comparing the patient's previous logs to their current log

Comparing the patient's previous logs to their current log appropriately evaluates the patient's attainment of their self-identified goals by comparing them with their outcomes. Addressing how the patient can properly check their glucose levels would be a step in assessing skill, not evaluating attainment of a self-identified goal. Asking the patient what they want to gain from improved monitoring is involved in goal setting and planning, a step that would have been completed before they implemented the plan to use the app. Recording the patient's log records in the patient chart is a process of documentation, not evaluation.

68. B) The patient has recently experienced stress

A probable explanation for this patient's laboratory values is recent stress, such as that from their acute infection. Their glucose ranges are well above a target range and are higher than expected for the A1C. The glucose and the A1C values would be higher if their diabetes was uncontrolled. However, they are not maintaining good control given that the glucose level is still elevated. If the patient recently started a new medication, the glucose would be more controlled and the A1C higher.

69. An older adult patient with type 2 diabetes and hypertension brings in their glucose and blood pressure log book. It is evident that they always check their blood glucose once in the morning and their blood pressure in the afternoon after their walk. What would be an appropriate recommendation for change?

    A. Add an additional glucose check during the day, and do not change the blood pressure check

    B. Keep the morning blood glucose check, and change the blood pressure check to mornings before medications

    C. Add an additional glucose check during the day, and check blood pressure once in the morning and once in the evening

    D. Continue to check both blood sugar and blood pressure at the same time every day

70. Which is a prerequisite of pattern management?

    A. Intact cognitive function

    B. Good vision

    C. Good manual dexterity

    D. The ability to do complex math

(*See answers next page.*)

69. C) Add an additional glucose check during the day, and check blood pressure once in the morning and once in the evening
The patient should add a second glucose check during the day and take their blood pressure once in the morning and once in the evening. Checking blood glucose at a variety of key times during the day can provide more awareness about glucose control. Blood pressure can tend to vary during the day and be highest in the morning. Checking blood pressure twice a day (once in the morning and once in the evening) can provide more meaningful results.

70. A) Intact cognitive function
The prerequisites of pattern management are commitment to development of skills, intact cognitive function, sound self-care skills, and strong problem-solving skills. Good vision, good manual dexterity, and the ability to do complex math are not prerequisites.

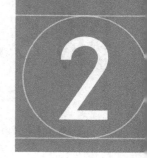

Interventions for Diabetes Continuum

2

1. A patient with type 2 diabetes is at a follow-up visit. They had established a goal for weight loss and are happy to see that they weight 7 lb less than their initial weight of 155 lb. They are 60 inches tall; their body mass index is 30.3. What is an appropriate recommendation for additional weight loss to achieve a sustainable weight loss goal? Guidelines are 5% - 10% Weight loss

A. 20 lb ⟵ 7 too much
B. 15 lb
C. 10 lb
D. 5 lb

155 lbs
×.10
15.50

155
7
148

155
-15
140

2. Which of the following is an incretin hormone stimulated by ingestion of food?

A. Bromocriptine
B. Neutral protamine hagedorn
C. Antithyroid peroxidase
D. Glucagon-like peptide 1

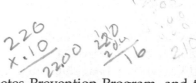

220
×.10
2200

220
2
16

210

3. A patient has completed the National Diabetes Prevention Program, and the diabetes educator provides feedback on their progress. They started the program at 220 lb and are now down to 204 lb and achieving 150 minutes of physical activity per week. According to the program's recommended goals, which feedback is most appropriate?

A. They met the weight loss goal but did not meet the physical activity goal
B. They did not meet the weight loss goal but met the physical activity goal
C. They met the goals for both weight loss and physical activity
D. They did not meet the goals for weight loss or physical activity

4. A patient with type 2 diabetes and high cholesterol has been instructed on ways to reduce fat in the diet and has attended a cooking class. They are taking medications to lower cholesterol and do not want to change drugs or increase dosage. Which action is appropriate for use as an intermediate outcome evaluation?

A. Clinical review of lipid measurements
B. Review of patient's food record
C. Having patient demonstrate ability to read food labels
D. Having patient list low-fat food choices

1. D) 5 lb
The patient needs to lose another 5 lb to achieve a sustainable weight loss goal. That would be achieving about an 8% weight loss. Current guidelines recommend sustaining at least a 5% to 10% weight loss to promote outcome improvements such as better A1C and glucose control. Weight loss of an additional 10 lb or more would be more than a 10% weight loss and is not a sustainable or realistic recommendation.

2. D) Glucagon-like peptide 1
Glucagon-like peptide 1 is made in the ileum and colon and provokes the secretion of insulin and the suppression of glucagon in response to incoming food. Bromocriptine is a dopamine agonist, which is proposed to function by stimulating the hypothalamus to affect insulin resistance associated with circadian cycles. Neutral protamine hagedorn, a long-acting insulin developed in 1946, is now known as NPH insulin. Antithyroid peroxidase is a thyroid auto-antibody that determines which patients are at a higher risk for thyroid autoimmunity.

3. C) They met the goals for both weight loss and physical activity
The National Diabetes Prevention Program's two major goals are achieving and maintaining a weight loss of 7% and performing 150 minutes of physical activity per week. This patient met both goals. The National Diabetes Prevention Program, established as a lifestyle intervention program by the Centers for Disease Control and Prevention, has established these two goals. The program recommends a 7% weight loss goal because it is feasible while still reducing the risk of diabetes. The goal of 150 minutes of physical activity is recommended in order to achieve an approximate 700-kcal per week expenditure from physical activity.

4. B) Review of patient's food record
Intermediate outcomes reflect on behavior changes, such as what would be documented on a food record. Lipid measurements are an objective post-intermediate outcome that is a desired clinical indicator of adherence to behavior change over a more consistent and longer time frame. Label-reading skills and listing low-fat food choices are most consistent with how to evaluate immediate outcomes in learning.

5. A patient with type 2 diabetes states that they are supposed to take 500 mg of metformin twice daily. However, they report abdominal discomfort when they take it. They state they are taking it first thing in the morning and just before bed. What is the most appropriate initial recommendation?

   A. Switch to a liquid version of metformin
   B. Take the doses with breakfast and dinner
   C. Discuss discontinuing the medication with their healthcare provider
   D. No recommendation is needed, but advise that symptoms will abate

6. A young adult patient with type 1 diabetes is missing insulin more often after getting a new job and a new apartment. In adjusting to their busy schedule, they often lose track of time and skip meals or miss an insulin dose. The diabetes educator discusses several strategies to manage their diabetes with the patient. At a follow-up assessment 3 weeks later, which skill would show that the patient is achieving an immediate outcome to their barriers?

   A. Demonstrates using smartphone apps for reminders
   B. Successfully demonstrates insulin administration
   C. Shows a trend of improving glucose in their log book
   D. States a plan for managing missed doses and treating hypoglycemia

7. The Dietary Guidelines for Americans 2015–2020 recommend reducing added sugars to less than what percentage of calories per day?

   A. 5%
   B. 10%
   C. 15%
   D. 20%

8. Measuring and documenting A1C evaluates which outcomes?

   A. Immediate
   B. Intermediate
   C. Post-intermediate
   D. Long-term

(See answers next page.)

5. B) Take the doses with breakfast and dinner

Taking their doses with meals is the best primary recommendation for this patient. Liquid versions of metformin would likely not change the adverse effects and only be beneficial with pill intolerance. Gastrointestinal adverse effects are very common, making discontinuation not a best recommendation. Although symptoms are known to abate, doing nothing is not appropriate because the patient is not taking the metformin with meals, which would help with the abdominal discomfort.

6. A) Demonstrates using smart phone apps for reminders

This patient's barrier is missing doses and skipping meals due to lack of time management. Their ability to demonstrate using smart phone apps for reminders is a way to evaluate an immediate outcome in overcoming that barrier. Being able to demonstrate dose administration, having a plan for handling missed doses, and treating hypoglycemia also evaluate immediate outcomes but do not address the patient's barrier. Reviewing log book records would evaluate an intermediate outcome to behavior change goals.

7. B) 10%

The Dietary Guidelines for Americans recommends consuming less than 10% of calories per day from added sugar. For example, a person on a 2,000-kcal daily diet should limit added sugars to no more than 200 calories. The Dietary Guidelines for Americans 2015–2020 states that the 10% target is based on food pattern modeling and national data. Although no recommended limit for sugar intake has been established, overall intake of calories and a healthy food pattern should be considered. A limit of 5% of calories per day from added sugars is likely to be too restrictive. For most calorie levels, there are not enough calories available after meeting food group needs to consume 15% or 20% of calories from added sugars and still stay within calorie limits.

8. C) Post-intermediate

Measuring A1C evaluates post-intermediate outcomes. Clinical measures such as A1C, lipids, blood pressure, and body mass index evaluate post-intermediate outcomes of behavior changes. Immediate outcomes include evaluating direct learning of knowledge, skills, and barriers. Intermediate outcomes comprise evaluating engagement in the desired behavior change, such as monitoring and being active. Long-term outcomes are assessed at follow-up visits to evaluate perception of quality of life and health status.

9. A patient with type 2 diabetes wants to understand why they have extremely high triglyceride levels. Which of the following explanations is most appropriate?

    A. "The glucose in your blood turns into triglycerides when storage depots for glucose are full."
    B. "You are most likely eating too much protein."
    C. "Your insulin resistance causes your body to be unable to properly use glucose for fuel, creating triglycerides."
    D. "Your diabetes has caused kidney damage, which makes it impossible for the kidneys to filter fat out of the blood as they should."

10. A patient is prescribed a sodium-glucose linked transporter-2 (SGLT2) inhibitor as additional oral therapy for type 2 diabetes. For which of the following side effects should the certified diabetes educator prepare the patient?

    A. Gastrointestinal symptoms
    B. Hypoglycemia
    C. Weight gain
    D. Increased urination

11. A 27-year-old pregnant patient presents at 25 weeks of gestation to be tested for gestational diabetes. They have eaten breakfast before the visit. Which of the following is the most appropriate plan of care?

    A. The patient meets criteria for testing and can proceed with a two-step 50-g oral glucose tolerance test (OGTT)
    B. The patient meets criteria for testing and can proceed with a one-step 75-g OGTT - fasting
    C. The patient meets criteria for testing and can proceed with a one-step 100-g OGTT 2nd part
    D. The patient's pregnancy is not far enough along to be tested and they should come back in a month 24-28 wks

9. C) "Your insulin resistance causes your body to be unable to properly use glucose for fuel, creating triglycerides."

Insulin resistance makes the body unable to properly use glucose for fuel, and the unused glucose builds up in the blood. As the level of glucose in the blood rises, increased fatty acid and triglyceride synthesis as well as inhibition of lipoprotein lipase cause the blood level of lipids to rise. Triglycerides are not correlated to any storage capacity; they are an effect of metabolic dysfunction. Carbohydrates are more closely correlated to triglyceride levels than are proteins. The kidneys have no significant impact on fat metabolism.

10. D) Increased urination

SGLT2 inhibitors work to decrease glucose by increasing glucose excretion; therefore, increased urination can be expected. SGLT2 inhibitors have additional side effects of low blood pressure, urinary tract infections, genital infections, and keto-acidosis. SGTL2 inhibitors are not associated with significant gastrointestinal distress or hypoglycemia. Additionally, SGLT2 inhibitors often support weight loss, not weight gain.

11. A) The patient meets criteria for testing and can proceed with a two-step 50-g oral glucose tolerance test (OGTT)

Testing for gestational diabetes by performing an OGTT is a standard of care for pregnancy. A two-step 50-g OGTT can be performed on a patient who has not fasted and can be followed by a 100-g OGTT if the test results are 130 mg/dL or higher (cutoff ranges vary from 130 to 140 mg/dL). The patient had not fasted; therefore, a 75-g one-step OGTT would not be recommended. Starting with a 100-g OGTT is also not standard practice because it is the second part of the two-step 50-g OGTT. All pregnant patients, regardless of risk factors, should be tested at 24 to 28 weeks of gestation; waiting another month is not recommended.

12. A patient is diagnosed with type 2 diabetes and is suffering from visual disturbances. They wonder if they should see an eye doctor for glasses. Which of the following is the best advice to give them?

    A. "Get an appointment as soon as possible with an eye doctor to correct your vision immediately."

    B. "An immediate dilated eye examination is recommended, but the blurred vision is likely a result of the high blood sugar and may improve with glycemic control."

    C. "Blurred vision should resolve within 2 to 3 months, but an eye examination is recommended if it does not resolve."

    D. "The blurred vision will likely improve within weeks; an eye exam would not likely be beneficial."

13. A patient has been taking an alpha glucosidase inhibitor (Acarbose) for 3 months since their diagnosis 6 months ago. Their A1C level is 7.8%. They reported frequent flatulence and diarrhea, so their doctor discontinued their metformin 3 months ago. Additionally, the patient has not been able to lose weight as desired. Which of the following plans of care is best to recommend for this patient?

    A. They can continue the current treatment but need to intensify their diet and lifestyle interventions

    B. They are should start a new dual-therapy treatment, such as a dipeptidyl peptidase-4 (DPP4) and a sodium-glucose linked transporter-2 (SGLT2) inhibitor

    C. They can continue current treatment but they need to have insulin initiated

    D. They need to go back to using metformin with the dose titrated carefully to relieve their gastrointestinal side effects

14. An adult patient is newly diagnosed with diabetes. The patient comments that they enjoy an occasional drink with dinner. What would be a pertinent education point regarding alcohol?

    A. Educate about the benefits of abstaining from alcohol

    B. Recommend moderation of one drink a week

    C. Educate about the risks for hypoglycemia

    D. Suggest reducing meal carbohydrates

(*See answers next page.*)

12. B) "An immediate dilated eye examination is recommended, but the blurred vision is likely a result of the high blood sugar and may improve with glycemic control."

Elevated glucose aggregates in the lens of the eye and leads to changes in the shape of the lens, causing visual disturbances. Blurred vision may improve within weeks, but care guidelines recommend a dilated eye exam at the time of diagnosis of type 2 diabetes to screen for undiagnosed diabetic eye disease. Recommending an eye appointment to correct the vision as soon as possible is not appropriate; time should be allowed for the resolution of hyperglycemia. An eye exam is recommended at time of diagnosis as well as annually for diabetic eye disease screening regardless of blurred vision resolution. Eye exams are a beneficial component to diabetes care.

13. B) They are should start a new dual-therapy treatment, such as a dipeptidyl peptidase-4 (DPP4) and a sodium-glucose linked transporter-2 (SGLT2) inhibitor

Guidelines from the American Association of Clinical Endocrinologists recommend dual therapy for diabetes if a patient's A1C level remains above 7.5% in 3 months. The alpha glucosidase inhibitors have only modest A1C efficacy and have gastrointestinal side effects. Continuing the patient''s current treatment is not an appropriate recommendation since it is ineffective. A possible change could be dual therapy of a DPP4 and an SGTL2 inhibitor. The SGLT2 inhibitor can also help with weight loss. Diet and lifestyle interventions alone will not be effective enough. Initiating insulin is an option but should be reserved for when the A1C is higher than 9.0%. Restarting metformin as monotherapy would probably not achieve desired goals despite recommendations to titrate the medication to relieve gastrointestinal side effects.

14. C) Educate about the risks for hypoglycemia

Current recommendations recognize the risks and need for education relating to the connection between alcohol intake and hypoglycemia. It is important to educate the patient about the risk of delayed hypoglycemia, especially if they are taking insulin or insulin secretagogues. Current recommendations do not necessarily warrant abstaining, and moderation is defined as one drink per day for women and two drinks per day for men. Reducing meal carbohydrates could further increase the hypoglycemia risk.

15. A 7-year-old patient is to have an oral glucose tolerance test (OGTT). Which of the following is an appropriate glucose load for them?

   A. 0.9 g/kg of body weight up to a maximum of 38 g of glucose
   B. 1.3 g/kg of body weight up to a maximum of 60 g of glucose
   C. 1.75 g/kg of body weight up to a maximum of 75 g of glucose
   D. 2.75 g/kg of body weight up to a maximum of 115 g of glucose

16. A patient with type 2 diabetes has been successful with achieving a goal of losing 35 lb in 6 months. What would be the next step to recommend?

   A. Support weight maintenance with a very-low-calorie diet and meal replacements
   B. Recommend a plan that supports a 500- to 750-kcal deficit for 3 more months
   C. Modify the diet to have an additional 20% restriction in fat and carbohydrates
   D. Provide support for weight monitoring and continuing diet and exercise

17. A patient newly diagnosed with type 2 diabetes asks for a diet plan suggestion to help manage their diabetes. Which specialized diet program is the most appropriate to suggest?

   A. Atkins
   B. South Beach
   C. Vegan
   D. DASH (Dietary Approaches to Stop Hypertension)

18. Basal insulin has been initiated for a patient with type 2 diabetes who is seeing the diabetes educator for a 1-month follow-up. The patient's glucose records for the past week show bedtime averages of 142 mg/dL and morning glucose averages of 84 mg/dL. The patient states that they walk before dinner and adds that dinner is sometimes late and less than 2 hours before bedtime, so the patient does not eat anything else after dinner. What would be an appropriate recommendation?

   A. Decrease the basal insulin
   B. Eat more at dinner
   C. Have a bedtime snack
   D. Stop walking before bedtime

(See answers next page.)

15. C) 1.75 g/kg of body weight up to a maximum of 75 g of glucose

The appropriate glucose load for a 7-year-old patient before an OGTT is 1.75 g/kg of body weight up to a maximum of 75 g of glucose. A fasting 75-g test has become an accepted researched standard for OGTT according to the American Diabetes Association and World Health Organization diagnostic criteria. The glucose loads of 0.9 g/kg of body weight, 1.3 g/kg of body weight, and 2.75 g/kg of body weight would not be likely to yield accurate results.

16. D) Provide support for weight monitoring and continuing diet and exercise

Initial intervention for those ready to begin weight loss requires an individualized plan of calorie reduction that works with their current food preferences and lifestyle. This patient needs support for weight monitoring and continuing diet and exercise. They have achieved their short-term goal and need a comprehensive weight maintenance program. A very-low-calorie diet meal replacement plan is an initial aggressive weight loss plan that needs close supervision. Modifying the diet further should continue to be individualized. General calorie reduction, not specifically just from fat and carbohydrates, can be similarly effective.

17. D) DASH (Dietary Approaches to Stop Hypertension)

The DASH diet is shown to be an effective eating pattern for the management of type 2 diabetes. The Atkins and South Beach diets have a focus on high-protein distribution and low carbohydrate, but they are not currently recognized as evidence-based, well-studied diets for diabetes. A vegan diet includes no animal products, which is not necessarily appropriate for diabetes management.f

18. A) Decrease the basal insulin

A consistent record of a greater than 30 mg/dL difference between bedtime and morning glucose levels indicates a possible need to reduce the basal insulin, usually by 10%. Eating more at dinner would mostly affect the patient's bedtime glucose, not the morning glucose. A bedtime snack would be a more appropriate recommendation if the patient had a lower bedtime glucose. A recommendation to stop walking is not likely to be beneficial; walking is not vigorous enough exercise to produce delayed hypoglycemia.

19. An adult patient newly diagnosed with type 2 diabetes asks the diabetes educator for advice about whether they should go on disability. The patient has been out of work for other reasons but now is concerned that having diabetes will make it hard to find a job. What would be the appropriate response?

   A. The patient cannot be considered to have a disability until their diabetes gets worse
   B. The diabetes educator can write a referral to support the patient's employment
   C. The patient should look for certain safe jobs due to the diabetes
   D. Employers do not need to know the patient's medical condition when the patient is applying for jobs

20. According to the Centers for Disease Control and Prevention (CDC), which of the following groups has the highest prevalence of diabetes?

   A. Native Americans
   B. Hispanic Americans
   C. Non-Hispanic Black Americans
   D. Asian Americans

21. A patient diagnosed with type 2 diabetes wonders why their glucose remains high when they feel that they have not eaten anything to increase their levels. Fasting glucose records reveal an average range of 150 to 175 mg/dL. What is the most likely cause?

   A. Generalized insulin resistance
   B. B-cell autoimmune destruction
   C. Too many carbohydrates eaten in the evening
   D. Decreased kidney function

22. A patient says that they are determined to achieve an A1C level of less than 7%. Which of the following is the best response?

   A. "Why not aim for 6.5%?"
   B. "What are your plans to achieve this?"
   C. "What do you want to try next if you can't get your A1C below 7%?"
   D. "Don't you think that we should try to get your cholesterol down, too?"

(See answers next page.)

19. D) Employers do not need to know the patient's medical condition when the patient is applying for jobs

Employers are not legally able to ask about health history while considering hiring and before a position is offered. Employers can request medical evaluation once an offer has been extended. Under the Americans with Disabilities Act of January 2009, all individuals with diabetes are considered to have a disability. This protects against discrimination but does not suggest an inability to be employed. A letter of referral is not sufficient and will not help with applications. However, an expert healthcare professional familiar with the patient may have to provide an assessment if questions of medical fitness arise. A formerly common belief was that diabetes should restrict individuals from certain jobs. This "blanket ban" practice is inappropriate.

20. A) Native Americans

According to the CDC, 15.1% of U.S. Native Americans have diabetes. In comparison, 12.1% of Hispanic Americans, 12.7% of non-Hispanic Black Americans, and 8.0% of Asian Americans have diabetes.

21. A) Generalized insulin resistance

Generalized insulin resistance, which leads to increased hepatic glucose production in the fasting state, suggests significant insulin resistance. Significant postprandial hyperglycemia in type 2 diabetes does not suggest a more significant insulin secretory defect, such as B-cell destruction. For some people, eating too few carbohydrates rather than too many carbohydrates in the evening causes a rebound effect of fasting hyperglycemia the following morning. Decreased kidney function often leads to hypoglycemia, not hyperglycemia.

22. B) "What are your plans to achieve this?"

Once the diabetes educator and the patient have reached an agreement about a general goal, the educator should ask the patient what they would like the target to be and how they would like to get there. If the patient has determined that their goal is an A1C level of less than 7%, the diabetes educator should not try to convince them to lower it further. If the patient is not able to change their level through lifestyle modification alone, they can discuss other options at an agreed-upon date (e.g., in 3 months or 6 months). To ask what the patient will try next implies an assumption that they are likely to fail. It is imperative that the patient be the one to choose the focus. Instead of telling the patient to tackle all possible goals at once, it is important to help them focus on one or two areas where the most advantage can be gained.

23. An adult patient is lean, presents with autoantibodies to islet cell components, and has developed manifestations of complete insulin deficiency with increasing insulin requirements. The patient most likely has which condition?

    A. Type 1 diabetes
    B. Type 2 diabetes
    C. Latent autoimmune diabetes of adulthood (LADA)
    D. Maturity-onset diabetes of the young (MODY)

24. Which statement regarding insulin is true?

    A. Insulin increases the transport of glucose into adipocytes
    B. Insulin stimulates the breakdown of glycogen
    C. Insulin decreases whole-body protein anabolism
    D. Insulin decreases mobilization of free fatty acids with fasting

25. An adult patient with type 2 diabetes has some retinopathy and neuropathy but is stable and in good health otherwise. The A1C is 7.1%. The patient is compliant with medications and glucose monitoring. When should the patient return for a follow-up A1C test?

    A. In 1 month
    B. In 3 months
    C. In 6 months
    D. In 1 year

26. A diabetes educator gives a guest lecture on diabetes pathophysiology to a class of medical students who have just returned from a lunch break. As the students digest their lunches, which concept would be ideal for the educator to emphasize in the lecture?

    A. Glucose production in the liver
    B. Proteolysis in the muscle
    C. Lipolysis in the adipose tissue
    D. Lipogenesis in the liver

(See answers next page.)

23. C) Latent autoimmune diabetes of adulthood (LADA)
Studies suggest that LADA develops from genes associated with both type 1 and type 2 diabetes coexisting in the patient, with signs and symptoms as experienced by this patient. Type 1 diabetes usually presents with insulinopenia before age 20 years. Type 2 diabetes patients usually are older than 30 years at diagnosis, are obese, and have relatively few classic symptoms. MODY is the term used to define a type of early-age diabetes that is associated with a gene mutation and presents as atypical diabetes.

24. A) Insulin increases the transport of glucose into adipocytes
Insulin increases the transport of glucose into adipocytes. Insulin stimulates glycogen synthesis, not breakdown, and maintains or stimulates whole-body protein anabolism in the presence of adequate plasma amino acids. With prolonged fasting, the plasma insulin concentration decreases and allows for increased, rather than decreased, mobilization of free fatty acids, which drives hepatic ketogenesis and results in ketosis.

25. C) In 6 months
As part of routine care, the American Diabetes Association recommends that A1C be tested at least two times a year for patients with type 2 diabetes who are meeting treatment goals and who have stable glycemic control. The A1C test should be performed quarterly for patients who have had a change in therapy and/or who are not meeting glycemic goals. Sooner point-of-care testing would be appropriate when considering or reviewing treatment changes. Waiting 1 year is not recommended.

26. D) Lipogenesis in the liver
In the fed state, glucose uptake and glycogen synthesis occur in the liver, sustained protein synthesis occurs in the muscle, and lipid synthesis occurs in the adipose tissue. Glucose production in the liver, proteolysis in the muscle, and lipolysis in the adipose tissue all occur in a low-insulin (fasted) state.

27. What is an appropriate food choice to treat mild hypoglycemia?

    A. 2 tbsp peanut butter
    B. 6 (2½-in) graham crackers
    C. 1 oz slice cheese
    D. ½ cup regular soda

28. A patient with type 2 diabetes states that they want to be more engaged in meeting activity goals but need motivation. The diabetes educator asks, "What would make you feel more engaged, and how can you reward yourself for success?" Which component of a problem-focused intervention is the educator using?

    A. Constructing a problem definition
    B. Collaborative goal setting
    C. Collaborative problem-solving
    D. Contracting for change

29. A diabetes educator meets with a patient before discharge. During the discussion, the educator touches on how the patient will manage their diabetes when sick. Which statement by the educator is the most appropriate?

    A. "When feeling bad, don't take your oral medications until you eat and feel better."
    B. "Call your doctor if you cannot get your blood sugar levels below 300."
    C. "Drink adequate fluids to prevent dehydration."
    D. "Test your glucose at least every 6 hours when you are ill."

30. A patient voices concern that they are not sure they can afford food at the end of the month. The educator notes that the patient is taking metformin and glipizide. The patient provides a diet history of processed foods and excessive carbohydrates such as bread and pasta. How could the educator be most helpful in this scenario?

    A. Assist the patient by teaching them how to shop on a budget
    B. Consult a dietitian who can educate the patient about carbohydrates
    C. Recommend changing glipizide to sitagliptin
    D. Refer the patient to a community social worker

(See answers next page.)

27. D) ½ cup regular soda

A half-cup of regular soda is an appropriate amount and source of carbohydrates to treat mild hypoglycemia. The treatment for mild hypoglycemia entails consuming 15 g of carbohydrate (preferably in the form of glucose), waiting 15 minutes, and retesting; if blood glucose remains less than 70 mg/dL, another 15 g of carbohydrate should be consumed. The testing and treating should be repeated until the blood glucose returns to the normal range. If it is more than 1 hour until the next meal, an additional 15 g of carbohydrate should be added to maintain blood glucose in normal range. Six graham crackers is closer to 30 g of carbohydrate. Peanut butter and cheese contain primarily protein and fat, which would not be appropriate food choices in a hypoglycemic situation.

28. D) Contracting for change

Contracting for change is setting criteria for success and a strategy to track outcomes. Constructing a problem definition refers to taking the patient's problem and defining it. Collaborative goal setting occurs when an appropriate goal is negotiated. With collaborative problem-solving, barriers to goal attainment are identified, and strategies to achieve the goal are formulated.

29. C) "Drink adequate fluids to prevent dehydration."

A patient with diabetes who is sick should drink adequate fluids to prevent dehydration. The patient should always continue oral medications and call the physician if oral medications are not staying down. Blood sugar staying above 300 is too high; it is recommended that patients contact a doctor when sugars remain above 240. When the patient is ill, checking the glucose level every 2 to 4 hours is recommended.

30. D) Refer the patient to a community social worker

The patient's primary problem is food insecurity. Patients with food insecurities often need assistance in seeking local resources, and a social worker can help with this. While the patient's diet indeed needs attention, education about shopping on a budget and consulting a dietitian will likely not be helpful in correcting food insecurity. Medication changes would not be recommended; glipizide is low in cost compared with sitagliptin, has a relatively short half-life to reduce the risk of hypoglycemia, and is a reasonable option when the patient is experiencing food insecurity.

31. A 57-year-old patient who has had type 2 diabetes for 12 years was started on glargine 9 months ago. Blood sugars show that fasting glucoses are at target under 130 mg/dL. The diabetes educator is concerned because the patient continues to have difficulty achieving A1C control. Which treatment would be an appropriate next step?

   A. Initiate insulin lispro before the largest meal of the day
   B. Discontinue glargine and start insulin lispro three times a day before meals
   C. Initiate insulin neutral protamine hagedorn (NPH)/regular 70/30 twice a day with glargine
   D. Continue glargine, but increase the dose

32. A reactive to proactive care delivery system, self-management support, and decision support that is based on evidence-based care guidelines are all elements of which delivery system?

   A. Patient-Centered Medical Home
   B. Chronic Care Model
   C. Process mapping
   D. Unified Medical Language System

33. Which insulin has an onset of 30 minutes to 1 hour?

   A. 70% neutral protamine hagedorn (NPH), 30% regular
   B. 75% insulin lispro protamine (NPL), 25% lispro
   C. 50% NPL, 50% lispro
   D. 70% aspart protamine, 30% aspart

34. Postprandial glucose checking is especially useful for patients:

   A. Who are suboptimally adherent to diabetes management
   B. Who are willing and able to check one or two times per day
   C. Whose A1C is elevated but whose fasting glucose is on target
   D. Who have type 1 diabetes using physiologic insulin replacement programs

(See answers next page.)

31. A) Initiate insulin lispro before the largest meal of the day

Insulin lispro should be started and taken before the largest meal of the day (4 units or 10% of basal dose). Current recommendations are to add rapid-acting therapy to basal insulin, not to discontinue basal therapy. NPH/regular 70/30 is an option, but it would require discontinuing glargine. Increasing the dose of glargine would likely not be effective and could be a risk for fasting hypoglycemia; adding therapy is recommended when a patient has achieved a fasting blood glucose target.

32. B) Chronic Care Model

The Chronic Care Model, which was designed to improve the quality of diabetes care, is composed of six elements: delivery system design, self-management support, decision support based on evidence-based care guidelines, clinical information systems, community resources and policies, and health systems. The Patient-Centered Medical Home is a system design initiative for improving outcomes through improving coordination of primary care and team-based management. Process mapping is a system more likely to be used as a tool for quality improvement. The Unified Medical Language System integrates and distributes key terminology, classification and coding standards, and associated resources to promote creation of more effective and interoperable biomedical information systems and services, including electronic health records.

33. D) 70% aspart protamine, 30% aspart

The onset for 70% NPH, 30% regular is 30 minutes to 1 hour. Onsets for 75% NPL, 25% lispro; 50% NPL, 50% lispro; and 70% aspart protamine, 30% aspart are all less than 15 minutes.

34. C) Whose A1C is elevated but whose fasting glucose is on target

Postprandial glucose checking is especially useful for patients whose A1C is elevated but whose fasting glucose is on target. Postprandial checking is also useful for those who are using (or considering using) glucose-lowering medications that specifically target postprandial glucose. Postprandial checking can be used as an evaluation tool if someone is trying to make dietary and physical activity modifications. People who are suboptimally adherent to diabetes management might be willing to use sporadic checking. People who are willing and able to check one or two times per day do well with systematic testing. Individuals with type 1 diabetes using physiologic insulin replacement programs should use intensive daily monitoring.

35. A patient who has type 2 diabetes wishes to make lifestyle changes to help improve their health as it relates to their diabetes. What would be an appropriate SMART (specific, measurable, attainable, relevant, and timely) goal for this patient?

    A. "I will aim to eat more vegetables to get more fiber."
    B. "I will walk in the mall for 30 minutes four times a week."
    C. "I will lose 50 lb by the end of the month."
    D. "I will work harder to check my glucose more often."

36. What is an appropriate time to test for ketones?

    A. During times of emotional stress
    B. After strenuous exercise
    C. When experiencing hypoglycemia
    D. While treating an infection

37. For a pediatric patient with type 1 diabetes, blood glucose should be checked a minimum of how many times per day?

    A. One
    B. Two
    C. Three
    D. Four

38. An 80-year-old patient with diabetes who has a history of smoking, hypertension, and retinopathy is accompanied by their adult daughter to a medical office visit. The daughter mentions to the diabetes educator that her parent will be moving in with her. She has valid concerns that the patient is not able to care for themself. What is the most appropriate action?

    A. Teach the importance of eye screening
    B. Reinforce treatment goals and self-care
    C. Refer to a community social worker
    D. Identify any adaptations in meal planning

(See answers next page.)

35. B) "I will walk in the mall for 30 minutes four times a week."
Mall walking for 30 minutes four times a week is a SMART (specific, measurable, attainable, relevant, and timely) goal. The goals of eating more vegetables and working harder to check glucose more often are not specific or measurable. Losing 50 lb by the end of the month is not likely attainable.

36. D) While treating an infection
During an illness or infection is an appropriate time to test for ketones. Other recommended times to test for ketones include when glucose levels remain above 250 to 300 mg/dL and during pregnancy. Emotional stress is not a sole factor in deciding to test for ketones, although it can be a cause for glucose elevation. Ketones should be checked before exercise, not after, if glucose levels are elevated, especially for people with type 1 diabetes. Ketones are associated with hyperglycemia, not hypoglycemia.

37. D) Four
At a minimum, blood glucose should be checked before each meal and at bedtime. Additional tests, such as 2 hours after meals, overnight, and before and after exercise, may also be necessary for establishing tighter glycemic control.

38. D) Identify any adaptations in meal planning
The educator should discuss diet with the patient and their daughter to identify any necessary adaptations in meal planning. There are four identified times for diabetes self-management education: at diagnosis, annually, with new complicating factors, and upon transitions in care. Education during transitions of care should include identifying needed adaptations in self-management and identifying level of involvement, such as when discussing diet. Instruction on the importance of eye screening would be more typical for new diagnosis education. Reinforcing treatment goals should occur annually. Referrals to social workers are most likely to be included as part of assistance when there are new complicating factors.

39. A young adult patient with type 1 diabetes wants better glucose control after meals and complains of weight gain and dissatisfaction with their A1C level. Which hormone therapy is an appropriate treatment for the patient's needs?

    A. Amylin
    B. Cortisol
    C. Glucagon-like peptide 1 (GLP-1)
    D. Glucagon

40. An adult patient with type 2 diabetes is confused about the glycemic index. They have heard that it is a way to choose carbohydrates but do not know why. Which explanation is most appropriate?

    A. The glycemic index is only necessary when you are taking insulin
    B. The glycemic index is an old method of carbohydrate counting
    C. Low-glycemic index foods are absorbed more slowly than high-glycemic index foods
    D. The glycemic index helps determine the amount of sugar in a food

41. A 17-year-old patient with type 1 diabetes has increasing problems with the dawn phenomenon. What would be an appropriate intervention?

    A. Increase the evening meal insulin aspart
    B. Increase the morning dose of aspart
    C. Add neutral protamine hagedorn (NPH) to the evening insulin
    D. Decrease the bedtime insulin glargine

42. Which statement is true regarding thiazolidinediones?

    A. They support weight loss
    B. They have low risk for hypoglycemia
    C. They have gastrointestinal side effects
    D. They are expensive

(See answers next page.)

39. A) Amylin
Amylin is a glucoregulatory hormone, approved for type 1 diabetes, that is co-secreted with insulin; they act together to regulate post-meal glucose concentrations. Amylin is associated with greater feeling of satiety, delayed stomach emptying, and related weight loss. Cortisol, a steroid hormone secreted by the adrenal gland, makes fat and muscles cells resistant to the action of insulin and enhances the production of glucose by the liver. GLP-1 is an incretin hormone—not effective as a treatment for type 1 diabetes—that is released from the gut and lowers glucose in several ways, including increasing insulin secretion and reducing appetite and glucose absorption. Glucagon is made by the islet cells in the pancreas, signals the liver to break down glycogen stores, and helps to form new glucose units and ketones from other substances.

40. C) Low-glycemic index foods are absorbed more slowly than high-glycemic index foods
Low-glycemic index foods are absorbed more slowly than high-glycemic index foods. Glycemic index ranks carbohydrates by how quickly they absorb and raise blood sugar. Carbohydrate counting, not glycemic index, is often necessary when on insulin. Glycemic index is a ranking of glucose absorption, not carbohydrate content or sugar content.

41. C) Add neutral protamine hagedorn (NPH) to the evening insulin
NPH insulin should be added to the evening insulin. Dawn phenomenon is an early-morning increase in glucose related to hormone-related rises in blood sugar and insufficient insulin. NPH, an intermediate-acting insulin, is a possible solution given in addition to the patient's required insulin to treat the dawn phenomenon. Increasing aspart, a rapid-acting insulin, at the evening meal or morning dose would not be effective. Decreasing glargine, a long-acting insulin, would not be effective and could worsen the dawn phenomenon.

42. B) They have low risk for hypoglycemia
Thiazolidinediones have a low risk for hypoglycemia. They have additional considerations of weight gain, not weight loss. Side effects are edema and heart failure concerns, not gastrointestinal effects. Generally, this is a low-cost medication.

43. A 50-year-old patient with type 2 diabetes presents with low-density lipoprotein (LDL) 143 mg/dL and blood pressure 142/91 mmHg. Recently the patient has been trying to stop smoking. The patient is not currently taking anything for cholesterol. What treatment will most likely be prescribed?

    A. A moderate-intensity statin
    B. A moderate-intensity statin plus ezetimibe
    C. A high-intensity statin
    D. Lifestyle changes and no prescription

44. A patient with type 2 diabetes is 5 ft 2 in tall and weighs 172 lb. The patient wants to know what a realistic weight loss goal would be. What is an appropriate recommendation for the initial weight loss goal?

    A. 8 to 12 lb
    B. 17 to 22 lb
    C. 25 to 32 lb
    D. 34 to 43 lb

45. Which concept is defined as a "collaborative, goal-oriented style of communication with particular attention to the language of change" and should be considered when individualizing education plans?

    A. Patient empowerment
    B. Transtheoretical model
    C. Motivational interviewing
    D. Health belief model

46. Current goals for medical nutrition therapy for diabetes include which action?

    A. Promoting a carbohydrate-reduced diet that is higher in protein and healthy fats
    B. Emphasizing nutrient-dense carbohydrate sources that are high in fiber and minimally processed
    C. Providing a guided meal plan that uses carbohydrate counting
    D. Reducing risk of deficiencies by promoting dietary supplementation of vitamins and minerals along with a healthy diet

(See answers next page.)

43. C) A high-intensity statin

A high-intensity statin treatment should be recommended due to the patient's age and cardiovascular risk factors. A moderate-intensity statin treatment would be recommended for a person of the same age who has no additional cardiovascular risk factors. A moderate-intensity statin treatment plus ezetimibe would be appropriate for a person with atherosclerotic cardiovascular disesase risk that is considered very high and with an LDL of 70 or higher on a maximally tolerated statin dose. Recommending lifestyle changes and no prescription would be appropriate for individuals younger than 40 years with no cardiovascular risk factors.

44. A) 8 to 12 lb

An appropriate initial weight loss goal for this patient is 8 to 12 lb. An initial weight loss of 5% is needed for many overweight or obese individuals with type 2 diabetes to achieve beneficial outcomes in glycemic control, lipids, and blood pressure. Clinical benefits are progressive, however, and more intensive weight loss goals may be appropriate for some.

45. C) Motivational interviewing

Motivational interviewing is a collaborative, goal-oriented style of communication that is beneficial when creating individualized education plans. Patient empowerment is similar to motivational interviewing but focuses more on supporting the patient's ability to discover and master self-care responsibility. The transtheoretical model provides a framework for the process of behavior change and has six stages ranging from pre-contemplation to termination. The health belief model is about understanding the reasoning behind behaviors and behavior change.

46. B) Emphasizing nutrient-dense carbohydrate sources that are high in fiber and minimally processed

There is no single ideal dietary distribution of calorie amounts of carbohydrates, fats, and proteins for people with diabetes. However, reducing carbohydrate intake for individuals with diabetes has demonstrated the most evidence for improving glycemia. Carbohydrate choices should come from nutrient-dense sources. Carbohydrate counting is less of a generalized goal and is supported as recommended education for those on intensive insulin regimens. There is little evidence to support general recommendations for dietary supplementation of vitamins and minerals.

47. A patient is 32 years old, has type 2 diabetes, and weighs 185 lb. The patient is generally healthy and has no complicating factors. They would like to know how much protein they should consume. What is the patient's minimal recommended amount per day?

A. 50 g

B. 67 g

C. 84 g

D. 100 g

48. What is the glycemic load of a piece of cornbread, which has a glycemic index of 110 and contains 30 g of carbohydrate?

A. 132

B. 82

C. 66

D. 33

49. A third-grade teacher has a new student in class who has known type 1 diabetes. What type of document would be best for the teacher to ensure is available as a plan of care?

A. A 504 Plan

B. An Individualized Education Plan (IEP)

C. Both a 504 Plan and an IEP

D. Neither a 504 Plan nor an IEP

50. An older adult patient with hypertension and high cholesterol is newly diagnosed with type 2 diabetes. The patient is a retired accountant and states that a sedentary life has "caught up" with them. The patient knows they need to exercise and eat better but does not know where to start. What education plan to address healthy eating objectives would be most appropriate for this patient?

A. Teach carbohydrate counting

B. Provide instruction on reading food labels

C. Explain the healthy plate model

D. Guide a menu-planning activity

(See answers next page.)

47. B) 67 g

The minimal recommended dietary allowance is 0.8 g protein/kg body weight, making the patient's minimum recommended protein intake 67 g/day (185 [lb] ÷ 2.2 = 84 kg; 84 x 0.8 = 67). The 50 g/day is below the minimum recommended protein intake. The American Diabetes Association (ADA) states that research is inconclusive regarding the ideal amount of dietary protein to optimize glycemic management and that protein intake goals should be individualized based on current eating patterns. Thus, the patient may choose to consume 84 g/day or 100 g/day, but the minimal recommended amount per day is 67 g.

48. D) 33

The glycemic load of a piece of cornbread is 33. Glycemic load is calculated by multiplying the glycemic index number of a food by the number of grams of carbohydrate in a serving and then dividing that number by 100: 110 x 30 = 3,300. 3,300 ÷100 = 33. The other results are incorrect using this formula.

49. B) An Individualized Education Plan (IEP)

The correct answer is an IEP. The IEP includes specific goals and requirements related to the student's learning goals and provisions for diabetes care. Any diabetic student who qualifies for services under the Individual with Disabilities Education Act is also covered by Section 504, so there is no need for two separate plans. An IEP is specific to each student, so it would be most appropriate for a new student, while a 504 Plan outlines the ways in which the school will ensure safety, fair treatment, and equal access to education for students with disabilities.

50. C) Explain the healthy plate model

The best place to start for this patient is the healthy plate model. Key features of the healthy plate model are that it is simple and does not require extensive explanation. It is a good place for the patient to start learning about healthier eating. Carbohydrate counting, reading food labels, and a menu-planning activity are more appropriate for someone who already feels comfortable with healthy eating basics but wants to develop further skills in food choices.

51. Which advice is most appropriate for the parents of a 3-year-old child with type 1 diabetes?

    A. Allow the child to help with glucose checks
    B. Use a reward system to encourage involvement
    C. Teach the child how to recognize the onset of hypoglycemia
    D. Have the child participate in food choices

52. A patient with type 2 diabetes wants to be more active but has a sedentary desk job. The patient's goal is to begin walking during lunch breaks and on weekends and to aim for 30 minutes each for 5 days out of the week. According to the current American Diabetes Association (ADA) recommendations, what additional advice is appropriate for this patient?

    A. Aim for 180 minutes of walking in a week
    B. Aim for 60 minutes of walking every day
    C. Interrupt periods of sitting every 30 minutes
    D. Interrupt periods of sitting every 60 minutes

53. A patient newly diagnosed with type 2 diabetes has demonstrated compliance with a treatment plan of lifestyle modifications and metformin for the last 3 months with fair success. However, at the last checkup, the patient's A1C had increased and is not at target after 3 months of therapy. What is an appropriate intervention for this patient?

    A. Reinforce lifestyle and carbohydrate control
    B. Add a glucagon-like peptide 1 (GLP-1) receptor
    C. Stop the metformin and initiate a sulfonylurea
    D. Add a meal-time rapid-acting insulin

54. Which condition is included in Stage 1 of the three stages of type 1 diabetes?

    A. Overt hyperglycemia
    B. Dysglycemia
    C. Normoglycemia
    D. No autoantibodies

(See answers next page.)

51. A) Allow the child to help with glucose checks

Even at a young age, a child with type 1 diabetes should be learning self-management. A 3-year-old may not be able to perform their own glucose checks but should be encouraged to watch and help. A child would need to be older to understand the reinforcement of a reward system, identify hypoglycemia, and participate in food choices. When a child is 3 years old, rewards are often not understood, and hypoglycemia symptoms are not apparent, so it is the responsibility of the parent to be aware and alert to those symptoms. A 3-year-old child would likely not have the cognitive ability to make healthy, appropriate food choices.

52. C) Interrupt periods of sitting every 30 minutes

Per current ADA recommendations, the patient should interrupt periods of sitting every 30 minutes. Current guidelines recommend a weekly goal of 150 minutes of physical activity, not 180 minutes. Sixty minutes of daily activity is the recommendation for children and adolescents. Breaking up sitting every 60 minutes is not frequent enough according to ADA recommendations.

53. B) Add a glucagon-like peptide 1 (GLP-1) receptor

Adding a GLP-1 receptor would be in line with current recommendations for adding therapy, thereby assisting in lowering the patient's A1C. Reinforcing lifestyle and carbohydrate control would likely not provide a benefit since compliance has already been demonstrated. Combination therapy is recommended, so stopping metformin is not necessary. Adding basal insulin, not rapid-acting insulin, could be a dual therapy option. Adding a meal-time rapid-acting insulin would be appropriate after further demonstration that A1C goals are not met after intensifying therapy.

54. C) Normoglycemia

Type 1 diabetes has been classified into three stages to serve as a framework for future research and regulatory decision-making. Stage 1, which includes normoglycemia, is believed to be an early stage that includes autoimmunity and multiple autoantibodies while being presymptomatic. Overt hyperglycemia is seen in Stage 3, and dysglycemia occurs in Stage 2. Stages 1 and 2 show autoantibodies . In Stage 3, autoantibodies may become absent.

55. When asked about home foot care, a patient reports doing nightly foot soaks and then applying lotion liberally to the feet. What would be the best response?

    A. Soaks are beneficial but be sure to keep water temperature cool
    B. Feet need to stay damp to absorb the moisturizer
    C. Routine foot soaks should be avoided
    D. Be sure to get lotion between the toes

56. What percentage of current body weight represents an effective amount of weight loss to reduce the risk of developing type 2 diabetes?

    A. 5% to 10%
    B. 10% to 15%
    C. 15% to 20%
    D. 20% to 25%

57. An adult patient with type 1 diabetes has increasing A1C values. Glucose levels are often above 250. The patient admits to skipping insulin injections, especially at work, and wants to change this behavior. The patient claims to work long hours and never get a break. The patient says, "My boss is so strict I am afraid to ask for a break or longer lunch." Which instructional strategy will be most helpful for this patient?

    A. Role-play different situations at work
    B. Provide handouts on ways to be more organized
    C. Discuss the importance of insulin adherence
    D. Suggest a medication reminder app

58. A 54-year-old patient with prediabetes says they understand that weight loss is a goal for managing their condition. When asked about their plan and goals, the patient states, "My goal is to lose 20 pounds." What is the diabetes educator's best follow-up question about this patient's stated goal?

    A. How is that goal realistic?
    B. How will that be achieved?
    C. Why just 20 pounds?
    D. How long will it take?

(See answers next page.)

55. C) Routine foot soaks should be avoided

Proper foot care includes routine washing of feet, but routine foot soaks should be avoided to maintain proper hygiene. Temperature regulation is important in any water environment, including showers, to avoid scalding. Feet must be dried thoroughly. Lotion is good for feet except for the area between the toes, which can be an area for fungus growth and should be kept dry.

56. A) 5% to 10%

A weight loss of 5% to 10% of current body weight would be effective to reduce the risk of developing diabetes type 2. The National Diabetes Prevention Program has established a goal of 7%, and research shows that weight loss as little as 5% to 10% of total body weight can reduce one's risk for developing type 2 diabetes. Weight loss above 10% is likely to be unfeasible.

57. A) Role-play different situations at work

Role-playing a variety of situations at work will help this patient actively learn, share, and explore options at work. The patient understands the importance of insulin, and disorganization is not a primary issue, so a discussion and handouts are not helpful. A medication reminder app could be helpful but does not address the patient''s concerns about their manager or the lack of breaks.

58. B) How will that be achieved?

Asking how the patient will lose the weight can lead to more discussion about steps and objectives to help the patient realize the goal. Asking whether the goal is realistic requires more specifics before evaluating if it is achievable. Asking why the patient is limiting the goal to just 20 pounds does not create rapport and is not collaborative. Asking how long it will take can be a way to set measurable goals, but it does not support discussion of the actions needed to achieve the goal.

59. An overweight patient is struggling to plan a diet for type 2 diabetes. By how much should the patient reduce their calorie intake?

    A. 125 to 250 kcal/day
    B. 250 to 500 kcal/day
    C. 500 to 750 kcal/day
    D. 750 to 1000 kcal/day

60. Which term refers to the process of reviewing evidence to determine the value or worth of something, such as education?

    A. Documentation
    B. Evaluation
    C. Assessment
    D. Quality improvement

61. Which factor will be included when evaluating a diabetic child's psychosocial adaptation?

    A. School attendance
    B. Child care plans
    C. Health insurance
    D. Major life events

62. Which learning objective should a level 1 educator be able to provide on a direct patient care level?

    A. Knowledge of basics
    B. Facilitating behaviors
    C. Evaluating outcomes
    D. Creating action plans

63. Which of these is a low-glycemic index food?

    A. Watermelon
    B. Pineapple
    C. Green peas
    D. Whole-wheat bread

(See answers next page.)

59. C) 500 to 750 kcal/day
The patient should reduce calorie intake by 500 to 750 kcal/day. This amount provides a weekly calorie deficit that would promote a 1- to 1.5-lb weight loss per week. Lower recommendations may not produce desired outcomes, and higher recommendations may be difficult to achieve or be too restrictive for this patient's sufficient daily energy requirements.

60. B) Evaluation
Evaluation is the process of reviewing evidence to determine the value or worth of an item or action. Documentation is a process that provides the data or evidence. Assessment is the careful process of collecting the relevant data to document and to be used in evaluations. Quality improvement is the process of using evaluations for continued development of processes and efficiency.

61. A) School attendance
School attendance can be a psychosocial risk factor for poor diabetes control and could be included when evaluating improvements or changes in psychosocial adaptation. Child care, health insurance, and major life events are more family-related risk factors, not psychosocial risk factors.

62. A) Knowledge of basics
A level 1 educator should be able to provide a knowledge of basics. There are three levels of practice. Level 1 educators are knowledgeable healthcare professionals but lack broad-based experience in diabetes as a specialty. Level 2 educators are advanced in diabetes-related knowledge and skills beyond basic professional skills. It is common to find level 2 educators facilitating behaviors with patients. Level 3 educators have achieved an expert level of practice in diabetes. This level of skill allows for evaluating outcomes and creating action plans at both patient and program levels.

63. C) Green peas
Green peas are a low-glycemic index food. Watermelon is a high-glycemic index food, and both pineapple and whole-wheat bread are medium-glycemic index foods.

64. Which instructional method would be most effective for a patient just starting insulin?

   A. Print materials
   B. Audiovisual aids
   C. Role-playing
   D. Demonstration and teach back

65. Which action can be considered a behavioral objective?

   A. Recording glucose levels in a log book
   B. Recognizing high sodium content on a food label
   C. Evaluating a menu for carbohydrate content
   D. Describing steps to treat hypoglycemia

66. Which statement best defines a learning objective?

   A. An intended change in behavior based on newly obtained knowledge or skills
   B. Meeting a level of sufficient knowledge to allow one to perform necessary skills
   C. The principal guide and focal point for education on necessary knowledge and skills
   D. A set of knowledge or skills desired to be met after education on necessary skills

67. Which activity is not among the seven self-care behaviors in the American Association of Diabetes Educators (AADE) framework in patient care education and goal setting?

   A. Being active
   B. Taking medication
   C. Collaborating
   D. Healthy coping

(See answers next page.)

64. D) Demonstration and teach back

Demonstration and teach back, such as demonstrating use of a glucometer or insulin injection, is the most effective instructive method to specifically enhance skills. Having the patient teach back the information ensures understanding. Print materials are best to provide hands-on resources and reinforce information already taught or not able to be covered in the presentation. Audiovisual aids can enhance learning and understanding but not necessarily skill. Role-playing is an activity that allows for group exploration and discussion.

65. A) Recording glucose levels in a log book

Recording glucose levels in a log book is a planned behavior. Recognizing sodium content, evaluating for carbohydrate content, and describing steps to treat hypoglycemia are more appropriate as learning objectives than as a learned knowledge or skill.

66. D) A set of knowledge or skills desired to be met after education on necessary skills

A learning objective is best defined as a set of knowledge or skills desired to be met after education. Behavioral objective is best defined as an intended change in behavior. Outcome is demonstrating a level of sufficient knowledge. A goal is the big picture, or principal guide, that drives the purpose behind education.

67. C) Collaborating

Collaborating is not among the seven self-care behaviors in the AADE framework in patient care education and goal setting. The seven behaviors are healthy eating, being active, monitoring, taking medication, problem-solving, healthy coping, and reducing risk.

68. An adult patient with type 2 diabetes has been working on their goal to quit smoking so they do not feel winded when walking. The patient says that the previous week was hard. The goal was to cut back to one cigarette a day, but some days they had two or more cigarettes. The patient still wants to quit smoking by the end of the month and believes they can do it. What is the diabetes educator's best question to evaluate the next steps in the patient's progress?

A. How would you rate your success or progress?
B. Do you feel the end of the month is still realistic?
C. Have you been able to walk more since cutting back?
D. Do you want to continue or change your goal?

69. A 58-year-old patient with type 2 diabetes has an increased A1C, from 7.4 to 9.5. The patient states that they are a new grandparent and have a "crazy" schedule now that they are helping their daughter and son-in-law with the baby. This schedule causes the patient to eat differently and skip taking medications more often than before. What is the best strategy for addressing this patient's environmental barrier to self-care goals?

A. Explore their reasons for not caring for themselves over others
B. Acknowledge their concerns and create a list of options
C. Seek understanding of why they perceive their life as "crazy"
D. Discuss their expectations and suggest a family meeting

70. An adult patient with type 2 diabetes wants to lose 10 pounds over the next 3 months. Which of the following is the most appropriate recommendation for implementation?

A. Refer the patient to the clinic's weight loss support group
B. Have the patient bring their weight log to each visit to review their progress
C. Discuss how often the patient exercises and what they eat
D. Have the patient write down what they desire from weight loss

(See answers next page.)

68. D) Do you want to continue or change your goal?
The educator should ask if the patient wants to continue or change the goal. Next steps would be to evaluate whether the goals should be changed, continued, or added to. Asking about success evaluates the patient's own assessment of the current goal. Discussing time frame and expected outcomes is a further collaborative assessment in evaluating a goal. Both are important in developing decision-making skills but are not specific to considering next steps.

69. B) Acknowledge their concerns and create a list of options
The patient's barrier is time and schedule, an environmental barrier. Acknowledging their concerns and creating a list of options is the best strategy for tackling environment-based barriers. Other options may be more appropriate for personal or interpersonal behaviors, such as barriers due to beliefs or relationship conflicts.

70. A) Refer the patient to the clinic's weight loss support group
The patient should be referred to the clinic's weight loss support group. Implementation includes providing an environment to achieve a desired goal and can include collaboration with others, as in a weight loss support group. The six process standards for diabetes education are assessing, goal setting, planning, implementation, evaluation, and documentation. A weight log is part of evaluation. Discussing the patient's lifestyle patterns (exercise, diet) is part of assessment. Writing down what the patient desires from weight loss is part of the discussion during planning.

71. A 6-year-old patient has had type 1 diabetes since age 2 years. The parents report that the patient cooperates well when they check the glucose levels. The parents want to encourage the patient's independence and ask about the next learning step. What is an appropriate instructional method and plan for this child based on this assessment?

    A. Play a game with the patient to teach the how to treat hypoglycemia
    B. Demonstrate insulin injection and have the patient demonstrate back
    C. Discuss the importance of maintaining parental involvement
    D. Role-play with parents on situations allowing more independence

72. A young adult patient with type 1 diabetes with a new insulin pump is following up on a previous session covering carbohydrate counting and carbohydrate-to-insulin ratio. The patient can identify carbohydrate foods, count the carbohydrates in a menu item, and describe when they need to adjust their pump, and they have kept a new log book with food intake, activity, and glucose levels. Which of these skills was a behavioral objective?

    A. Being able to identify carbohydrate foods
    B. Being able to count the carbohydrates in a menu item
    C. Being able to describe when to adjust his pump
    D. Being able to keep a daily record in a log book

73. Which factors should be documented as part of the goal-setting process?

    A. Patient's attitudes and health beliefs
    B. Recommended strategies and interventions
    C. Referrals, resources, and communication
    D. Treatment objectives and expected outcomes

74. An adult patient who has had type 2 diabetes for 2 years has completed a series of diabetes education classes and returns for an annual evaluation. What is an appropriate action step for this patient's annual assessment?

    A. Demonstrate monitoring and discuss when to test blood glucose
    B. Develop and support personal strategies for healthy coping
    C. Support efforts to sustain initial behavior changes
    D. Provide education for others now involved in patient's care

(See answers next page.)

71. C) Discuss the importance of maintaining parental involvement

It would be appropriate to discuss the importance of maintaining parental involvement. Age 6 years is too early to begin to encourage total independence, and parental involvement needs to be reinforced and supported. Skills to treat hypoglycemia and insulin injection skills are generally recommended at about age 10 to 12 years. Role-playing with parents might encourage the parents to place too much responsibility on the child at this age.

72. D) Being able to keep a daily record in a log book

Keeping a log book is a measurable and observable goal consistent with a behavioral goal. Identifying and counting carbohydrates and recognizing when to adjust the insulin pump are more consistent with knowledge-based goals, or learning objectives.

73. D) Treatment objectives and expected outcomes

Treatment objectives and expected outcomes are documented in the goal-setting process. Goal setting is a next step after assessment that would include documentation of what is desired, or the expected outcome, from any treatment or intervention. Attitudes and beliefs would be included in the assessment. Referrals, resources, and communication would be included in the implementation.

74. C) Support efforts to sustain initial behavior changes

The appropriate action step is to support efforts to sustain initial behavior changes. A basic annual evaluation is a chance to assess and review successes and challenges, which includes a discussion in support of current efforts in self-management behaviors since the patient will have already made behavioral changes. Monitoring blood glucose demonstration would have been done at diagnosis. Developing and supporting personal strategies for behavior change and healthy coping is most appropriate when new complicating factors influence self-management. Providing education for others now involved in care is necessary only when there is a transition in care.

75. Which method is best to evaluate meter technique?

    A. Teach back
    B. Log book
    C. Patient demonstration
    D. Lab results

76. Which of the following is a benefit of continual glucose monitors (CGMs) for evaluating blood glucose records?

    A. Elimination of finger sticks
    B. Facilitation of understanding and use
    C. Support of treatment decision-making
    D. Reduction of risk from hyperglycemia

77. A diabetes education program manager realizes that even after several class sessions, many students are unable to correctly identify glucose goals when monitoring. What instructional plan would be appropriate for this educator to include in the next class?

    A. Address fears and attitudes toward finger sticks
    B. Provide log books for home glucose monitoring
    C. Review signs and symptoms of high and low glucose
    D. Demonstrate the use of a glucose meter in class

78. What is a key function of good documentation?

    A. Establishes a framework for motivation and rapport
    B. Specifies expected outcomes and behaviors
    C. Provides key information for decisions and outcomes
    D. Identifies the value and effectiveness of a process

79. A young adult patient with type 1 diabetes brings their glucose meter and log book for review. The log book lists the blood sugar, when the blood sugar was taken, and when the meals were eaten. What other information would the diabetes educator need to fully evaluate this log book?

    A. Food intake
    B. Symptoms
    C. Site used
    D. Control tests

(See answers next page.)

75. C) Patient demonstration
Meter technique is a skill that would be best observed by the educator, so the patient would demonstrate how to use the meter. Teach back implies a patient's ability to verbally demonstrate learning, which would be more effective to evaluate understanding of learning points or medications but not skills such as use of a meter. A log book would support meter use but not specifically technique. Lab results would be a way to evaluate for discrepancies in meter results or records.

76. C) Support of treatment decision-making
CGMs can be a beneficial tool to support decisions on dosing of insulin, food intake, and activity planning. CGMs, however, are not meant to totally replace standard finger stick glucose monitoring. They can be complicated, and their use requires numeracy skills. CGMs are most often used to reduce the risk of and provide feedback on hypoglycemia, not hyperglycemia.

77. B) Provide log books for home glucose monitoring
Having a log book for home glucose monitoring would allow for further discussion of target goals and reinforce knowledge of general target goal recommendations. A quiz would imply an assessment of knowledge only when developing a plan for instruction and education. Addressing feelings about finger sticks and demonstrating in class would imply developing a plan of action based on assessment of attitudes and skills. Reviewing signs and symptoms of high and low glucose is a separate knowledge set from creating target goals.

78. C) Provides key information for decisions and outcomes
Documentation provides key information for decisions and outcomes. Assessment is a preliminary step that establishes motivation and rapport. Goal setting outlines desired outcomes and behaviors. Evaluation identifies the value and effectiveness of a given process.

79. A) Food intake
The diabetes educator needs to know the food intake that corresponds to these measurements. The primary goal of a log book is to be a self-management tool. Decisions about self-care would be most useful if food intake, along with activity and medications, were included in the log book. Symptoms would be important to discuss if there were frequent instances of hypoglycemia but would not be instructive if medications, food, and activity were not understood. Site used is not absolutely necessary for the log book, but knowing the type of meter is important. Control tests can be a good tool for testing the accuracy of a meter, but they are not necessary for every use or for the log book.

80. A 32-year-old patient with type 2 diabetes and hypertension, a body mass index of 32, and a history of smoking is recovering from a heart attack. The patient states that they are ready to make some lifestyle changes. Which is an appropriate follow-up question to initiate developing goals?

    A. "What have you tried to change in the past?"
    B. "What barriers do you see in making changes?"
    C. "What do you expect from making changes?"
    D. "That is wonderful! What changes are possible?"

81. A patient with type 2 diabetes is overweight and inactive. The patient is confident that they can make changes and wants to start exercising to lose weight. A discussion of physical activity reveals that current activity is limited to household chores. The patient establishes a goal to increase walking by 30 minutes every week for the next 3 weeks and to keep an activity and weight log. At the 3-week follow-up, the patient reports some success, and the log book documents walks and weight. What diabetes self-management education (DSME) process was achieved by discussing physical activity for weight loss?

    A. Evaluation
    B. Assessment
    C. Planning
    D. Goal setting

82. A patient has type 2 diabetes and is a Vietnam veteran. They ask if they may be eligible for disability compensation. What would be an appropriate follow-up question?

    A. Have you been exposed to Agent Orange?
    B. Did you develop pancreatitis during your service?
    C. Did you eat army food for 2 consecutive years?
    D. Were you exposed to mustard gas testing?

83. A patient with type 2 diabetes is adding glyburide as an additional therapy to their metformin. What will the educator need to address with this patient regarding the medication changes?

    A. Reducing other medications such as metformin
    B. Importance of monitoring for edema
    C. Risks of hypoglycemia
    D. Likelihood of weight loss

(*See answers next page.*)

80. D) "That is wonderful! What changes are possible?"

Asking "What changes are possible?" opens a discussion toward goal setting by focusing on what could be possible or what the patient feels able to do. A helpful acronym about goal setting and individualizing goals is DARN: Desire, Ability, Reasons, and Need. Asking about past changes, barriers, and expected outcomes is most relevant after narrowing a goal and does not focus on the actual intent, which is a behavior change goal.

81. D) Goal setting

The patient achieved the DSME process of goal setting. Goal setting establishes a treatment area and expected outcomes. Goal setting was completed by deciding on physical activity as a treatment with the expected outcome of weight loss. Evaluation involves reviewing the patient's report of success and ability to keep a log book. Assessment would be the data collected at the beginning of the documentation. Planning would be the recommended intervention of walking and keeping an activity log.

82. A) Have you been exposed to Agent Orange?

Vietnam veterans with type 2 diabetes might be eligible for disability compensation from the Department of Veterans Affairs (VA) if they were presumed to be exposed to Agent Orange or other herbicides. In 2000, the VA added type 2 diabetes to the list of "presumptive diseases associated with herbicide exposure." Pancreatitis, consumption of army food, and mustard gas testing are not associated with the development of type 2 diabetes in Vietnam veterans.

83. C) Risks of hypoglycemia

The educator should advise the patient about the risks of hypoglycemia. This is due to glyburide being a sulfonylurea, which affects the pancreas by improving insulin secretion. Glyburide is a dual therapy addition, and dose correction is not necessary. Edema is a risk associated with thiazolidinediones. Potential for weight gain, not weight loss, exists with use of glyburide.

84. An adult patient with newly diagnosed type 2 diabetes needs instruction on how to inject insulin. They will go home with an insulin pen that uses 4-mm pen needles. What would be appropriate education?

    A. There is no need to pinch a skin fold for injections
    B. The patient can use only the abdomen for an injection site
    C. The patient needs to insert the needle at a 45-degree angle
    D. There is no need to prime the pen before injection

85. Which is the current recommendation regarding wrist monitors for blood pressure?

    A. Testing can be done without regard for exercise
    B. The arm needs to be below the level of the heart
    C. The test result should be adjusted for overestimation
    D. Use of wrist monitors is not recommended

86. Which of the following best describes how alcohol can be a contributing factor to causing diabetes?

    A. Alcohol reduces the body's sensitivity to insulin
    B. Alcohol causes the muscles to release more glucose
    C. Alcohol causes liver inflammation, impacting glucose metabolism
    D. Alcohol reduces the kidney's ability to filter sugar

87. According to the SMART method of goal setting, which is the best example of a goal?

    A. "I will eat green vegetables at lunch every day starting tomorrow."
    B. "I will contact pharmaceutical assistance programs to see if they can help me afford my meds."
    C. "I will walk for 30 minutes five mornings a week starting on Monday."
    D. "I will make my appointment for a yearly physical on Monday morning."

88. A 32-year-old patient with type 2 diabetes states that they are getting married and would like to become pregnant within a year. They provide a medication list that includes metformin and atorvastatin. What is the correct recommendation?

    A. Continue both the metformin and the atorvastatin
    B. Continue the metformin and discontinue the atorvastatin
    C. Discontinue the metformin and continue the atorvastatin
    D. Discontinue both the metformin and the atorvastatin

(See answers next page.)

84. A) There is no need to pinch a skin fold for injections

There is no need to pinch a skin fold to make this injection. A needle with a length that small does not need a skin pinch to ensure delivery to subcutaneous fat. Rotation of all sites (abdomen, thigh, buttock, and arm) is recommended. A 90-degree angle is generally recommended. The pen should always be primed to ensure proper dose administration.

85. D) Use of wrist monitors is not recommended

Wrist monitors are generally inaccurate and not recommended since they yield less reliable readings. Testing recommendations include avoiding exercise for at least 30 minutes before the reading. The arm should be placed at heart level, not below. Overestimation can occur due to cuff size or sleeve constriction; however, there are no current recommendations on adjustments, only using proper technique.

86. A) Alcohol reduces the body's sensitivity to insulin

Alcohol reduces the body's sensitivity to insulin. There is evidence that alcoholism is a contributing cause of diabetes in three ways: reducing insulin sensitivity, causing chronic pancreatitis, and being a source of excessive calories that can cause obesity.

87. C) "I will walk for 30 minutes five mornings a week starting on Monday."

The best example of a goal is, "I will walk for 30 minutes five mornings a week starting on Monday." "SMART" stands for "specific, measurable, achievable, realistic, and time-bound." A goal to eat green vegetables is not specific or measurable. Plans to contact assistance programs and to make a physical exam appointment are steps toward potential SMART goals.

88. B) Continue the metformin and discontinue the atorvastatin

The patient should continue the metformin but discontinue the atorvastatin. Patients who could become pregnant should avoid statins, and metformin is considered safe in pregnancy.

89. An older adult patient on insulin therapy comments that their insulin can look clumpy. The patient states that they store their insulin in the freezer to keep it fresh. What is the appropriate response?

    A. The patient can freeze insulin for up to 3 months
    B. Once the patient thaws insulin, they should not refreeze it
    C. The patient needs to thaw insulin in the refrigerator
    D. The patient should stop freezing their insulin

90. A patient with type 2 diabetes complains of weight gain. Examination shows that they have lower extremity edema. Which medication are they most likely taking?

    A. Glimepiride
    B. Metformin
    C. Rosiglitazone
    D. Liraglutide

91. Which drug used to treat diabetes is most associated with weight gain?

    A. Metformin
    B. Glipizide
    C. Dapagliflozin
    D. Exenatide

92. A patient asks how being obese might cause diabetes. Which response is most appropriate?

    A. Obesity contributes to insulin resistance and proteins that affect glucose metabolism, which may lead to diabetes
    B. Obesity does not actually cause diabetes; rather, they are comorbidities
    C. Oxygen and nutrients are diverted to the extra fat tissue, requiring blood vessels to pump more blood to this tissue
    D. Fat deposits build up in the arteries, reducing blood flow to the heart

93. Which podiatry condition, sometimes found in patients with diabetes, includes symptoms of a red and swollen foot that is hot to touch?

    A. Bunions
    B. Hammer toes
    C. Charcot foot
    D. Foot ulcers

(See answers next page.)

89. D) The patient should stop freezing their insulin

The patient should stop freezing their insulin. Freezing temperatures will break down the insulin and it will not work well to lower blood sugar.

90. C) Rosiglitazone

The patient is taking rosiglitazone, which is a thiazolidinedione. Thiazolidinediones are usually combined with other medications and should be discontinued if the patient gains weight or retains fluid as evidenced by edema of the lower extremities. Glimepiride is a sulfonylurea, and adverse effects can include hypoglycemia and weight gain, but without the edema. Metformin, a biguanide, and liraglutide, a glucagon-like peptide 1 (GLP-1) agonist, are more commonly associated with gastrointestinal adverse effects and have been shown to cause weight loss.

91. B) Glipizide

Glipizide has been associated with weight gain. Metformin, dapagliflozin, and exenatide are more likely to be weight neutral or support weight loss.

92. A) Obesity contributes to insulin resistance and proteins that affect glucose metabolism, which may lead to diabetes

Obesity contributes to insulin resistance and proteins that affect glucose metabolism, which may lead to diabetes. It is not true that obesity is simply a comorbidity of diabetes; it may cause diabetes by contributing to insulin resistance. Obesity does cause oxygen and nutrients to be circulated to fat tissue, but this is a cause of high blood pressure, not diabetes. With obesity, fat deposits may build up in the arteries, resulting in reduced blood flow to the heart. However, this is a cause of heart disease, not diabetes.

93. C) Charcot foot

Charcot foot causes redness and swelling and makes the foot hot to the touch. Bunions cause the big toe to angle toward the second toe, causing the joint at the base of the big toe to protrude. Hammer toes occur when the toes become arched in either direction. Foot ulcers may present as a callus or thick skin and may have discharge.

94. A 27-year-old patient with type 1 diabetes wants to exercise more. They have a history of moderate nonproliferative retinopathy. What is the most appropriate recommendation for this patient?

    A. Continue routine eye exams with no need to limit exercise
    B. Avoid heavy lifting and strenuous exercises
    C. Choose walking, as it is the best exercise considering these conditions
    D. Have an exercise stress test before starting exercise

95. A patient with type 2 diabetes reports having a desk job. They have gained 15 lb in the last year and feel it is due to inactivity. The plan is to provide an exercise prescription. What is the most appropriate topic to include in the prescription?

    A. The type of exercise they should consider
    B. The amount of weight loss desired from exercise
    C. The types of carbohydrates to consume around exercise
    D. The goals of glucose monitoring when increasing exercise

96. The Dietary Approaches to Stop Hypertension (DASH) diet can decrease blood pressure by up to how much?

    A. 7 mmHg
    B. 14 mmHg
    C. 21 mmHg
    D. 28 mmHg

97. Which supplement is often used to support treatment of hyperlipidemia?

    A. Milk thistle
    B. Ginseng
    C. St. John's wort
    D. Fish oil

98. A 26-year-old pregnant patient has been diagnosed with gestational diabetes mellitus (GDM). The patient is concerned about the health of the fetus. Which complication is most associated with GDM?

    A. Microcephaly
    B. Tetralogy of Fallot
    C. Macrosomia
    D. Caudal dysgenesis

(See answers next page.)

94. B) Avoid heavy lifting and strenuous exercises

Avoiding heavy lifting and strenuous exercise is the most appropriate recommendation for this patient. Due to this patient's advanced retinopathy, considerations of safety with exercise should be made; so, while routine eye exams are necessary, it is not true that there is no need to limit exercise for this patient. Walking is a safe, low-impact exercise to recommend, but other low-impact exercises such as stationary bike riding and lane swimming are also appropriate. It is important to include that heavy lifting and strenuous exercise should not supplement these activities. A stress test can be a consideration, but current criteria recommend stress testing after age 30 with type 1 diabetes and retinopathy. A stress test would not be a first recommendation for a patient who is 27.

95. A) The type of exercise they should consider

It is appropriate to discuss the type of exercise the patient will do. An exercise prescription should include the type of exercise or activity, the defined workload (such as weight or speed), the duration and frequency of the program, intensity guidelines (such as target heart rate and estimated rate of perceived exertion), any specific precautions, the recommended progression, and activities for special situations (such as business travel or vacation). The exercise prescription does not need to include a specific weight loss goal, types of carbohydrates, or goals for glucose monitoring.

96. B) 14 mmHg

The DASH diet can decrease blood pressure by up to 14 mmHg. Eating a diet that is rich in whole grains, fruits, vegetables, and low-fat dairy products and that is low in saturated fat and cholesterol can lower blood pressure by up to 14 mmHg. The DASH diet can lower blood pressure by more than 7 mmHg but not typically by as much as 21 mmHg or 28 mmHg.

97. D) Fish oil

Fish oil is a complementary medicine product commonly used to lower cholesterol; it is a natural supplement that can support a decrease in triglycerides. Milk thistle is more often used and studied for its effectiveness in treating hepatic disease. Ginseng is commonly used for immune support and is studied more for glucose control than cholesterol control. St. John's wort is used for psychiatric disorders such as depression and anxiety rather than hyperlipidemia.

98. C) Macrosomia

Macrosomia, or large birth size, is the complication most associated with GDM. Microcephaly, tetralogy of Fallot, and caudal dysgenesis are all congenital birth defects associated with infants of those with pre-existing diabetes. Congenital malformations are not highly associated with GDM.

99. Which exercise choice is an example of a vigorous-intensity activity?

   A. Jumping rope
   B. Doubles tennis
   C. Ballroom dancing
   D. Bicycling 8 mph

100. What is ectopic fat?

   A. Fat that is stored in the liver, muscle, and pancreas
   B. Fat that is stored under the skin
   C. Fat that is in smaller stores in the neck, collarbones, and deep in the skin
   D. Fat that is stored in the abdomen

(See answers next page.)

99. A) Jumping rope

Jumping rope is considered a vigorous-intensity activity. Doubles tennis, ballroom dancing, and bicycling 8 mph are all examples of moderate-intensity activities. Vigorous-intensity activity is physical activity done on a scale relative to an individual's personal capacity, usually 17 to 19 on a scale of 1 to 20.

100. A) Fat that is stored in the liver, muscle, and pancreas

Ectopic fat is stored in the liver, muscle, and pancreas. Ectopic fat may block the signal that insulin sends to glucose transporters. Liver fat is a better predictor of metabolic dysfunction than visceral fat. Subcutaneous fat is fat stored under the skin. Brown fat is often in smaller stores along the neck and collarbones; it is often associated with burning calories and providing heat. Fat stored in the abdomen is more commonly known as visceral fat.

Disease Management

1. A patient with type 2 diabetes is admitted at 8 a.m. for elective surgery. They report that they took their medications, including metformin, the day before. They have been NPO (nothing by mouth) since midnight and placed on blood glucose checks every 4 hours. Immediately before surgery, their blood glucose is 85 mg/dL. After surgery, they are given clear liquids, and their blood glucose is 163 mg/dL. Which statement is true about the patient's condition before and after surgery?

   A. The metformin should have been withheld
   B. The 4-hour glucose checks are too far apart
   C. The patient's presurgery glucose is below target
   D. The patient's postsurgery glucose is above target

2. A patient with type 2 diabetes is admitted for treatment of an abscess. They are on oral medications at home, which are withheld at admission. Their glucose levels are consistently above 180 mg/dL fasting and after meals. What would be an expected plan of care?

   A. Start an intravenous insulin protocol
   B. Order scheduled neutral protamine hagedorn (NPH)/regular insulin
   C. Initiate a sliding scale protocol
   D. Begin a basal plus bolus correction plan

1. A) The metformin should have been withheld

The patient's metformin should have been withheld. Perioperative inpatient guidelines specify a recommendation to withhold metformin at least 24 hours before surgery to reduce the risk of lactic acidosis. Glucose checks 4 to 6 hours apart are appropriate. Target ranges for the perioperative period are 80 to 180 mg/dL, so both pre- and postsurgery glucose levels are in range.

2. D) Begin a basal plus bolus correction plan

A basal plus bolus correction plan is an appropriate recommended standard of care for noncritical patients. An intravenous insulin protocol can be appropriate in the critical care setting. NPH/regular insulin has been shown to increase hypoglycemia risk in the inpatient setting. A sliding scale is not encouraged as a sole glycemic control plan of care.

3. An adult patient with type 1 diabetes presents to the clinic with an A1C level of 11.5% and a history of not using insulin or a meal plan. The certified diabetes educator overhears the physician telling the patient that any A1C level higher than 7.0% can lead to complications and that they will need aggressive treatment and better compliance. The patient becomes visibly upset and states that a level of 7.0% is impossible for them. Which of the following actions is the best way to support the patient's education needs?

   A. Agree with the physician that the patient must achieve an A1C of 7.0% to see a decrease in the risk of complications

   B. Educate the physician that achieving an A1C of less than 7.0% should be avoided because it results in severe hypoglycemia, which can further harm the patient

   C. Educate the physician that although intensive diabetes therapy and compliance are necessary, setting a less restrictive A1C goal can still have good outcomes and result in better patient compliance

   D. Educate the physician that patients must achieve an A1C goal of 6.5% to see a decrease in the risk of complications

4. Standard 3 as defined by the National Standards for Diabetes Self-Management Education and Support (NSDSMES) refers to which aspect of program quality standards?

   A. Advisory board appointment and responsibilities in the program

   B. Established curriculum and assessment tool development

   C. Proper assessment and identification of target population

   D. Program staff development, responsibilities, and credentials

5. In response to an increase in admissions and readmissions related to diabetes, a large city hospital has assigned a taskforce to implement a diabetes quality improvement plan. A component of the improvement plan includes enhancing discharge information and education. Which healthcare professionals would be most important to recruit to implement the proposed changes and enhancements?

   A. Physicians

   B. Nurses

   C. Pharmacists

   D. Educators

(See answers next page.)

3. C) Educate the physician that although intensive diabetes therapy and compliance are necessary, setting a less restrictive A1C goal can still have good outcomes and result in better patient compliance
The Diabetes Control and Complications Trial (1993) provided evidence that intensive diabetes therapy is effective in reducing the risk of long-term complications. However, an important conclusion of the study was also that patients do not need to achieve an A1C level of less than 7.0% to see a reduction in the risk of complications; anything that is done to improve the A1C level is advantageous. It is true that the group receiving intensive therapy had a threefold increase in hypoglycemia, but hypoglycemia incidents decreased as the participants became more accomplished at using intensive insulin therapy. In the intensive group, three or more daily insulin injections were given, and an injection of regular insulin was administered before each meal. The patients, based on self-monitoring of blood glucose levels, modified the dosage of regular insulin as appropriate. An A1C level of 6.5% may be a goal for certain low-risk groups but can be indicative of hypoglycemia in certain high-risk groups that have highly variable glycemic control.

4. C) Proper assessment and identification of target population
There are currently 10 standards for the NSDSMES. Standard 3 relates to access, which would encompass proper assessment and identification of target populations. Standard 2 applies to external input to include establishment of an advisory board. Standard 6 covers meeting curriculum content. Standard 5 addresses program staff development and considerations.

5. B) Nurses
A valuable asset in patient education is nurses. Staff nurses are often charged with the responsibility to assess and address education needs. It would be meaningful to target, educate, and provide nurses with the resources they need to educate. Physicians, pharmacists, and educators will likely take a role in education; however, they will often have other responsibilities. For example, a physician or pharmacist may be more appropriate when targeting for development of protocols and medication safety. An educator will need to devote time to managing and overseeing larger education projects or be at multiple settings and are therefore not likely able to fully meet the needs of education as well as a nurse can in discharge planning.

6. A patient with hypertension and a body mass index of 40 presents to the clinic for a health screening exam. Their fasting plasma glucose level is 118 mg/dL. Which of the following is the most appropriate advice for the patient?

   A. "You should repeat a fasting plasma glucose test in a year."
   B. "You should get a glucose meter and occasionally test your glucose at home."
   C. "You should have a urine test to see if you are spilling glucose."
   D. "You should be considered for oral glucose tolerance testing."

7. At a 4-month follow-up visit, a 14-year-old patient with type 2 diabetes measures 5 feet 7 inches tall and weighs 195 pounds. They have a repeat blood pressure that is greater than the 90th percentile for their age, sex, and height. Their lipid profile is 89 mg/dL. They have joined a soccer team and the family has been working on dietary changes. What treatment recommendation should the diabetes educator anticipate?

   A. Initiate an angiotensin-converting enzyme inhibitor (captopril)
   B. Initiate a statin (lovastatin)
   C. Initiate both an angiotensin-converting enzyme inhibitor and a statin
   D. Encourage continuing lifestyle improvements only

8. Which technique is the most effective for teaching patients how to choose foods when eating out?

   A. Short lecture
   B. Self-assessment
   C. Case studies
   D. Role-playing

(See answers next page.)

6. D) "You should be considered for oral glucose tolerance testing."

The patient should be considered for oral glucose tolerance testing. A fasting plasma glucose level of 100 to 125 mg/dL is considered to be indicative of impaired fasting glucose. Anyone with impaired fasting glucose, especially if there are other risk factors such as hypertension and obesity, should be considered for an oral glucose tolerance test to assess postprandial glucose patterns. Repeating the glucose test in a year misses an opportunity for prevention. Current recommendations do not include either self-testing blood glucose or urine testing as criteria for diabetes health screening exams.

7. A) Initiate an angiotensin-converting enzyme inhibitor (captopril)

Starting an angiotensin-converting enzyme inhibitor such as captopril would be an appropriate treatment given that the patient's blood pressure is greater than the 90th percentile for age, sex, and height. Their lipid profile is below the recommended 100 mg/dL so a statin or dual therapy is not needed, according to recommendations. Encouraging lifestyle changes would be appropriate but may not be sufficient treatment in this case.

8. D) Role-playing

Role-playing is the most useful technique for reinforcing learning and exploring personal problems, such as ordering at restaurants, in an active manner. A short lecture would be more appropriate when imparting new information and providing knowledge important for patient self-care. Self-assessment is a good tool for helping patients recognize problems in diabetes self-management and identify solutions to those problems using their blood glucose records, food diaries, and exercise logs. In this case, the problem is already identified and needs to be further explored. Case studies provide an objective approach to learning but would probably not provide the application-based learning that would be most useful in exploring ways to problem-solve. Case studies are best used for planning and problem-solving when helping patients identify errors in methods they use to manage their diabetes.

9. A patient has type 2 diabetes. They tell the diabetes educator that they are confused about what their glucose goals should be 2 hours after meals. One physician told them that their goal should be 140 mg/dL, while another said that their goal should be lower than 180 mg/dL. Which of the following statements best explains the discrepancy?

   A. The second physician is using outdated American Diabetes Association (ADA) guidelines, and new guidelines recommend that 2-hour postprandial glucose be lower than 140 mg/dL

   B. The first physician is using outdated American Association of Clinical Endocrinologists (AACE) guidelines, and new guidelines recommend that 2-hour postprandial glucose be lower than 180 mg/dL

   C. The first physician is using the recommendations set by the AACE, and the second physician is using the recommendations set by the ADA

   D. Neither physician is correct; the patient should be primarily interested in keeping the A1C level lower than 7%

10. An elementary school child has been diagnosed recently with type 1 diabetes. Their parent, in a meeting with school representatives, voices concerns that the teacher will not allow students to have snacks in the classroom. Which response by the school representatives is appropriate?

    A. By law, the school has the right to limit snacks in the classroom

    B. The parent must obtain a written diagnosis and plan that documents required accommodations and instructions

    C. The school recognizes the parent's concerns and recommends relocation to a school better equipped to handle students with complicated health needs

    D. The school requires that the child eat all snacks in the nurse's office

11. Which of the following would most likely be included in continuous quality improvement (CQI)?

    A. Total billed hours

    B. Survey responses

    C. Cost of materials

    D. Marketing activity

(See answers next page.)

9. C) The first physician is using the recommendations set by the AACE, and the second physician is using the recommendations set by the ADA

The first physician is using the recommendations set by the AACE, and the second is using the recommendations set by the ADA. The ADA recommends an A1C level of less than 7%, a preprandial glucose level of 70 to 130 mg/dL, and a peak postprandial blood glucose level of less than 180 mg/dL. The AACE recommends an A1C level of less than 6.5%, preprandial glucose lower than 110 mg/dL, and 2-hour postprandial glucose lower than 140 mg/dL.

10. B) The parent must obtain a written diagnosis and plan that documents required accommodations and instructions

A 504 plan is an extensive plan that includes accommodations and care instructions for students with disabilities, including those with diabetes. This plan provides specific rights to the child and limits discrimination. To obtain a 504 plan, the parent must provide the school with documentation of the child's diagnosis and recommendations for accommodations from the child's physician. Schools do not have the legal right to limit snacks for a child who may require them for medical purposes. Recommending an alternative school based on a medical diagnosis is discriminatory. It would be disruptive to the class and to the student to insist that the child take all snacks in the nurse's office. Proper training of school staff is required.

11. B) Survey responses

Survey responses are a common way to collect data to assess an identified problem and aim to develop a CQI process/plan. Total billed hours are more common in a productivity report. Cost of materials would be appropriate in a budget. Any outreach would include marketing activity.

12. What would be an appropriate reading grade level for diabetes education materials to be used in classes and at the bedside?

    A. 3rd grade
    B. 6th grade
    C. 9th grade
    D. 12th grade

13. A 26-year-old patient is 15 weeks pregnant and has no risk factors for diabetes or symptoms of diabetes. When should they be screened for gestational diabetes?

    A. At 16 weeks
    B. At 24 weeks
    C. At 30 weeks
    D. Never; no need to be tested

14. A 27-year-old patient with gestational diabetes arrives at the clinic for a routine follow-up visit. Glucose logs show fasting glucose between 74 and 92 mg/dL and 2-hour postprandial glucose between 130 and 150 mg/dL. What would be appropriate feedback on the glucose record?

    A. The fasting glucose levels are too low
    B. The fasting glucose levels are too high
    C. The 2-hour postprandial glucose levels are within normal limits
    D. The 2-hour postprandial glucose levels are too high

15. A 79-year-old patient arrives in the ED with confusion, decreased alertness, lethargy, and poor appetite for several days. Lab results reveal glucose of 887, arterial pH of 7.4, trace ketones, and serum bicarbonate of 17 mEq/L. Which would be the most appropriate diagnosis and subsequent plan of care?

    A. The patient is in diabetic ketoacidosis (DKA) and requires fluids, insulin, and intravenous (IV) bicarbonate
    B. The patient is in DKA and requires fluids, insulin, and an electrolytes check
    C. The patient is in a hyperosmolar hyperglycemic state (HHS) and requires fluids, insulin, and IV bicarbonate
    D. The patient is in an HHS and requires fluids, insulin, and an electrolytes check

(See answers next page.)

12. B) 6th grade

Experts recommend that health education materials be written at a 6th grade level. Some believe that imposing a grade level too low is too limiting and can lead to poor cohesion. However, most health education materials are written at the 9th grade level or above, which may limit patient comprehension. Readability formulas, which usually assess the number of syllables per word, can help assess the complexity of written materials.

13. B) At 24 weeks

A gestational diabetes screening should happen at 24 to 28 weeks. According to the U.S. Preventive Services Task Force, screening before 24 weeks is not helpful, and screening after 24 weeks is later than necessary. All pregnant patients should be screened for gestational diabetes, regardless of their risk factors or symptomatology.

14. D) The 2-hour postprandial glucose levels are too high

The guidelines for gestational diabetes recommend keeping the 2-hour postprandial glucose at or below 120 mg/dL and 1-hour postprandial glucose at or below 140 mg/dL. Glucose at or below 95 mg/dL is recommended as a fasting goal.

15. D) The patient is in an HHS and requires fluids, insulin, and an electrolytes check

An HHS often presents with altered mental status and lab diagnostics that include glucose greater than 600 mg/dL, arterial pH greater than 7.3, zero to trace ketones, and serum osmolality greater than 320 mOsm/kg. DKA presents with varying mental state, glucose greater than 250 mg/dL, present ketones, variable serum osmolality, and serum bicarbonate less than 15 mEq/L. The patient meets the criteria for HHS, not DKA. Treatment for either requires aggressive fluid resuscitation, insulin, and monitoring of other electrolytes; bicarbonate is not required because there is no acidosis with HHS.

16. A patient with type 2 diabetes has applied for a job as a product delivery driver. The patient voices concern that the company is questioning their ability to drive because of their diabetes, and they believe this is discriminatory. Which statement is the most appropriate response to this patient?

A. "Having a diagnosis of diabetes is not reason enough to question your ability to drive."

B. "You must prove you are not taking insulin to qualify for any driving position."

C. "You obtained your license without medical evaluation, so you're at risk."

D. "Having diabetes does make you an unsafe choice for the company to hire."

17. An older adult patient with type 2 diabetes is admitted to the hospital ICU with urinary tract infection–related sepsis, hypotension, and respiratory failure. The patient's blood glucose levels have been between 218 and 289 mg/dL. The provider has orders to initiate insulin and routine glucose checks. Which glucose target range will most likely be recommended as a patient treatment goal when initiating this patient's insulin?

A. 110 to 140 mg/dL

B. 140 to 180 mg/dL

C. 180 to 210 mg/dL

D. 200 to 240 mg/dL

18. According to a consensus of the American Association of Clinical Endocrinologists and the American Diabetes Association, which statement is true concerning the use of non-insulin antihyperglycemic agents in the hospital setting?

A. These agents are typically not appropriate for most hospitalized patients who require therapy for hyperglycemia

B. These agents are appropriate for all patients with diabetes who have not experienced hypoglycemia in the past 72 hours

C. These agents should usually be given at a lower dose than they are taken at home

D. These agents should be given at the usual dose for anyone younger than 70 and should not be given to those older than 70 at any dosage

(*See answers next page.*)

16. A) "Having a diagnosis of diabetes is not reason enough to question your ability to drive."

Having diabetes is not enough reason to question a person's ability to drive, according to the American Diabetes Association's position statement on diabetes and driving. Taking insulin is also not enough of a reason to limit driving; exemption programs exist even for commercial drivers using insulin. Medical evaluation is a possible requirement upon a state's inquiry before licensure, but this varies across states and jurisdictions and is not always necessary. Safety concerns after episodes of hypoglycemia can also trigger a medical evaluation referral. A person with diabetes should not be discriminated against as an unsafe choice for hire simply for having a diabetes diagnosis.

17. B) 140 to 180 mg/dL

For the critically ill patient with persistent hyperglycemia, insulin therapy should be initiated at a threshold no greater than 180 mg/dL. Once insulin therapy has been started, a glucose range of 140 to 180 mg/dL is recommended for most critically ill patients. A target goal of 110 to 140 mg/dL may be appropriate in certain cases if more stringent goals do not confer hypoglycemia risk. Target goals of 180 to 210 and 200 to 240 mg/dL are often too high for effective treatment. According to the American Diabetes Association (ADA), more moderate glycemic targets (140–180 mg/dL) for critical care patients promote better outcomes and less hypoglycemia.

18. A) These agents are typically not appropriate for most hospitalized patients who require therapy for hyperglycemia

Non-insulin antihyperglycemic agents are not appropriate for most hospitalized patients who require therapy for hyperglycemia. Scheduled subcutaneous administration of insulin with basal, nutritional, and correction components is preferred for achieving and maintaining glucose control. Administration of non-insulin agents is allowed at times, per clinical judgment, but there are no current hypoglycemia, dose adjustment, or age criteria for inpatient administration.

19. An older adult patient with a history of diabetes has abdominal pain and is admitted to the hospital for observation. The patient is found to have a bowel obstruction and will be NPO (nothing by mouth). What would be the expected frequency of glucose testing?

    A. At least once every hour
    B. At least once every 2 to 4 hours
    C. At least once every 4 to 6 hours
    D. At least once every shift

20. An adult patient with type 1 diabetes is in the ICU for diabetic ketoacidosis and is being treated with an insulin drip infusion. The insulin drip is to be discontinued and the patient transitioned to subcutaneous insulin. What would the anticipated physician order be?

    A. Initiate basal insulin at 70% of the daily infusion rate 1 to 2 hours before the intravenous insulin is discontinued
    B. Initiate basal insulin at 60% of the daily infusion rate 1 to 2 hours after the intravenous insulin is discontinued
    C. Initiate basal insulin at 50% of the daily infusion rate immediately after the intravenous insulin is discontinued
    D. Initiate basal insulin at 100% of the daily infusion rate 1 to 2 hours after the intravenous insulin is discontinued

21. Which of the following factors would negatively impact the rapport and communication process between a patient and an educator?

    A. Perceiving the educator as educated and competent
    B. Feeling of being in an environment that supports expressing feelings
    C. Viewing the diabetes educator as having authority over care
    D. Recognizing that the educator allows silence during session conversations

(*See answers next page.*)

19. C) At least once every 4 to 6 hours

This patient's blood glucose should be monitored at least once every 4 to 6 hours. Intravenous insulin would require more frequent monitoring. Most shifts are 8 hours or longer, which would not be as appropriate for monitoring of glycemic control.

20. A) Initiate basal insulin at 70% of the daily infusion rate 1 to 2 hours before the intravenous insulin is discontinued

When transitioning intravenous insulin to subcutaneous insulin, guidelines recommend that basal insulin be initiated 1 to 2 hours before the intravenous insulin is discontinued, not after. A basal insulin dose of 60% to 80% is appropriate and shown to be effective.

21. C) Viewing the diabetes educator as having authority over care

Demonstrating authority can have a detrimental effect on communication. Being perceived as competent, providing a supportive environment, and allowing silence are strategies conducive to good communication.

22. A patient with a history of diabetes is admitted to inpatient care for a noncritical illness. Insulin therapy has been initiated due to persistent hyperglycemia. The patient generally has good intake at meals. Glucose ranges after insulin initiation have been between 142 and 174 mg/dL. Which statement is appropriate regarding the patient's glucose control?

    A. The patient is not meeting glucose goals of less than 130 mg/dL
    B. The patient is meeting target glucose ranges of 140 to 180 mg/dL
    C. The patient is above acceptable glucose ranges and may require insulin adjustment
    D. The patient is a little above acceptable glucose ranges, but this is permissible

23. All of these factors would be listed as provisions on the Individualized Education Plan (IEP) for a student with diabetes EXCEPT:

    A. How annual goals will be tracked
    B. Current levels of performance
    C. Any limitations in available services
    D. Standardized test-taking modifications

24. An older adult Spanish-speaking patient is admitted to the hospital and is newly diagnosed with type 2 diabetes. The patient's grandchild is in the room and says they can take any educational materials and explain them to the patient. What would be the most appropriate intervention?

    A. Provide a DVD in Spanish that the patient can take home
    B. Ask a nurse who speaks Spanish to help communicate with the patient
    C. Consult with an interpreter to assist with the education
    D. Agree to have the grandchild help with the education

25. What is the first approach the American Diabetes Association (ADA) would take when assisting in advocating for legal rights in a case that involves discrimination due to diabetes?

    A. Negotiate
    B. Educate
    C. Litigate
    D. Legislate

(See answers next page.)

22. B) The patient is meeting target glucose ranges of 140 to 180 mg/dL

According to consensus of the American Diabetes Association and the American Association of Clinical Endocrinologists, for the majority of noncritically ill patients treated with insulin, the target glucose range is 140 to 180 mg/dL. More stringent goals of less than 140 mg/dL may also be appropriate. Adjusting insulin is not required given that the patient's glucose is within acceptable ranges. Higher ranges may be permissible in terminally ill patients and patients with severe comorbidities, or in a care setting where frequent glucose monitoring is not feasible.

23. C) Any limitations in available services

Statements about limitations in services would not be included in the IEP for a student with diabetes. The IEP contains a statement of how the child's progress toward annual goals will be tracked. It also contains a statement of the present level of performance (including how the disability affects involvement and progress in the general curriculum); a statement of measurable annual goals, including benchmarks or short-term objectives; a statement of special education and supplementary aids and services to be provided; and a statement of modifications needed for the child to participate in district-wide tests or other assessments.

24. C) Consult with an interpreter to assist with the education

Consulting a trained medical interpreter would be the most appropriate approach to ensure that any education points as well as patient comments are correctly conveyed. Providing a DVD may be good follow-up material, but patient-specific education in the hospital must take place first. Asking a nurse to assist is not as ideal as a trained interpreter. Continuing the education with the help of the grandchild can result in miscommunication and put privacy at risk.

25. B) Educate

The first approach is to educate. The four steps of the ADA approach to legal rights are educate, negotiate, litigate, and legislate. The other steps follow education.

26. The head of diabetes education at a large clinic has been asked to organize information for a review of the program. A goal is to demonstrate that standards are being met. Which information should be included?

    A. Documentation of Medicare certification
    B. Strategies to promote health and behavior change
    C. The mission statement and goals of the program
    D. The program budget

27. A staff nurse is caring for an adult patient with diabetes who requires nutrition via a percutaneous endoscopic gastrostomy tube. The patient is currently on continuous feeds. The patient's glucose at 8:00 a.m. was 124 mg/dL. At what time should the nurse repeat a glucose check?

    A. 11 a.m.
    B. 1 p.m.
    C. 3 p.m.
    D. 8 p.m.

28. An adult diabetes education class includes participants acting out ordering food at a restaurant during the nutrition portion of the class. Which type of learning does this represent?

    A. Kinesthetic
    B. Visual
    C. Observational
    D. Verbal

29. Which factors are some of the curriculum content areas defined in the National Standards for Diabetes Self-Management Education?

    A. Pathophysiology of diabetes and treatment options, healthy eating, being active, and taking medication
    B. Goal setting, motivation, resolving family issues, and planning around holidays and special events
    C. Drinking responsibly, tobacco cessation, maintaining oral health, and obtaining financial assistance
    D. Foot and nerve health, use of tracking tools, stress reduction, and understanding health insurance

(See answers next page.)

26. C) The mission statement and goals of the program

National Standards for Diabetes Self-Management Education and Support has 10 total standards for a quality program. Organizational structure is one standard that would include demonstrating having a mission statement and goals. The other standards include advisory group information; target population information; having a coordinator, instructors, and a curriculum; demonstrating individual patient assessment; demonstrating a personalized follow-up plan; showing measurements of patient-defined goals and patient outcomes; and having continuous quality improvement. Meeting the standards is required to qualify for Medicare reimbursement; a certificate is not part of the standards. A budget is also not a specified part of the standards. Strategies to promote health and behavior change is a content area of diabetes self-management education that could fall under a curriculum standard but is not a specific standard for the program itself.

27. B) 1 p.m.

If a patient is receiving cycled enteral nutrition, continuous enteral nutrition, or parenteral nutrition, a good standard of care is to check every 4 to 6 hours. Therefore, the nurse should recheck the patient's glucose at 1 p.m. in order to meet that standard. Checking as early as 11 a.m. would not usually be necessary, and waiting beyond 6 hours would not lead to optimal glucose control.

28. A) Kinesthetic

Kinesthetic learning includes role-playing, which is learning by acting out the principle to be learned. Reviewing an illustration is an example of visual learning. Observational learning is a type of reflective learning. Watching the diabetes educator perform a blood glucose test is an example of observational learning. Learning by listening to a lecture is an example of verbal learning.

29. A) Pathophysiology of diabetes and treatment options, healthy eating, being active, and taking medication

The curriculum content areas include pathophysiology of diabetes and treatment options, healthy eating, being active, and taking medication. The other content areas are healthy coping, monitoring, reducing risk, and problem-solving and behavior change strategies. Goal setting, motivation, resolving family issues, holidays and special events, drinking alcohol, tobacco cessation, oral health, financial assistance, foot and nerve health, tracking tools, stress reduction, and understanding insurance are not included in the National Standards for Diabetes Self-Management Education, although they may be common topics in numerous other resources such as publications from the American Diabetes Association and the American Association of Clinical Endocrinologists.

30. The director of a diabetes program in a large health system reviews a report on the program's referral base. The report shows that many referrals stem from the local hospital, not from primary care providers. This factor often delays scheduling because of the need to communicate back to the primary care provider to approve the referral. What is an appropriate solution?

    A. Approach local hospital leaders to establish a better referral plan of action
    B. Delegate program employees to be assigned to the hospital to assist in referrals
    C. Complete a time study to fully assess concerns about delay before making changes
    D. Implement a community outreach plan that includes local primary care clinics

(See answers next page.)

30. D) Implement a community outreach plan that includes local primary care clinics

An appropriate solution is to implement a community outreach program to include local clinics, educating and reaching primary care clinics as a way to concentrate on the referring provider. Focusing attention on the hospital and its leaders and employees will likely not lead to desired changes and could stress resources. This is not a productivity issue, so a time study would not be pertinent.

Part II
Practice Exam and Answers
With Rationales

Practice Exam

1. A diabetes educator is aiming to improve a poorly attended diabetes self-management education program. The educator would like the program to be accredited and is meeting with a committee to determine planning. The committee would like to know which quality indicator will be targeted for accreditation. Which action is an appropriate quality improvement goal plan?

   A. Increase the participant show rate
   B. Decrease patient lab entry errors on the referrals
   C. Decrease the lipid values of the patients
   D. Increase the satisfaction of the patients

2. A diabetes educator presents a proposal for a diabetes education program to the clinic's administrative committee. The committee requests that the program's learning objectives be clearly stated. Which of the following is an appropriate learning objective for the program?

   A. To identify blood glucose goals
   B. To believe that diabetes can be managed
   C. To understand healthy meal planning
   D. To acknowledge the importance of exercise

3. An adult patient with type 2 diabetes states that they are having difficulty managing foods when eating out and at social events. Which would be the best teaching format for diabetes education for this patient?

   A. Booklets
   B. Web-based learning
   C. Discussion
   D. Role-playing activity

4. The parents of a 12-year-old patient with diabetes would like to meet with the child's appropriate school personnel to address creating an Individualized Education Plan. The parents discuss the request with the patient's teacher and mention that the teacher is the first person at the school that they have notified about the need for an Individualized Education Plan. Who else should the teacher recommend be involved in the discussion?

A. An attorney
B. The physical education teacher
C. A qualified occupational therapist
D. A qualified representative of the school district

5. A diabetes educator is developing a curriculum based on the AADE7 Self-Care Behaviors. In developing the curriculum, the educator wants to focus on the core behavior change topics. Which topic is the educator most likely to include?

A. Knowledge skills
B. Problem-solving
C. Smoking cessation
D. Weight loss

6. A patient with type 2 diabetes states that despite 3 months of diet and exercise, they have been unsuccessful in losing weight. The patient's body mass index remains higher than 30. Which medication is an appropriate treatment option?

A. Fluoxetine
B. Triamterene
C. Exenatide
D. Liraglutide

7. An 83-year-old patient with type 2 diabetes voices concern about moving in with their adult son, who does not know much about diabetes. What is an appropriate area of focus in the discussion?

A. Reinforce to the patient the importance of nutrition
B. Discuss strategies for risk reduction and prevention of complications
C. Screen the patient for depression and diabetes distress
D. Establish the patient's current skills of self-management

8. A nurse assistant is triaging a patient with diabetes at a local hospital. The nurse assistant knows this patient and is aware that the patient does not know much about diabetes care. What aspect of diabetes education is the nurse assistant qualified to give this patient?

   A. Importance of routine checkups
   B. Technique for injecting insulin
   C. Blood glucose monitoring schedules
   D. Ketone testing

9. A patient brings medications for review during an initial diabetes education assessment visit and is unable to specifically point out certain medications by name but refers to them by color and shape. Which issue may need further assessment when working with this patient?

   A. Health literacy
   B. Vision barriers
   C. Numeracy problems
   D. Reading literacy

10. An adult patient with an 8-year history of type 2 diabetes reports frequent and burning urination. A urine culture confirms a urinary tract infection. A review of medications shows atorvastatin, metformin, dapagliflozin, and lisinopril. For which medication does this patient need education on risk of urinary tract infections?

    A. Atorvastatin
    B. Metformin
    C. Dapagliflozin
    D. Lisinopril

11. A 9-year-old patient with type 1 diabetes is being seen for a routine visit. The patient's parent expresses concern because the child has too many hypo-glycemic episodes. What should the certified diabetes educator assess in the patient?

    A. Ability to demonstrate awareness of hypoglycemia at all times
    B. Ability to adjust insulin doses
    C. Ability to treat episodes when they occur
    D. Ability to recognize and report symptoms

12. A pregnant 24-year-old patient with type 1 diabetes presents their glucose records for evaluation. The records include only fasting glucose, after-dinner glucose because it is the biggest meal, and nighttime. Which ongoing plan is best for this patient's monitoring goals?

    A. Maintain the monitoring goals
    B. Monitor before the meal, not after
    C. Monitor before and after all meals
    D. Monitor at more varied times

13. An adult patient with type 2 diabetes has been working on improving adherence to self-monitoring. The patient provides a log with the following glucose measurements for the previous week. What does this log indicate that the patient should be evaluated for?

    - Sunday: Prebreakfast: 130 mg/dL
    - Monday: Postbreakfast: 225 mg/dL; bedtime: 69 mg/dL
    - Tuesday: Prebreakfast: 110 mg/dL; predinner: 185 mg/dL
    - Wednesday: Postbreakfast: 253 mg/dL
    - Thursday: Prelunch: 125 mg/dL
    - Friday: Prebreakfast: 116 mg/dL
    - Saturday: Postbreakfast: 216 mg/dL

    A. Prevention and awareness of hypoglycemia
    B. Changes to carbohydrate intake at breakfast
    C. Possible medication changes for fasting glucose levels
    D. Activity changes to lower predinner glucose levels

14. The diabetes educator follows up with a patient to review progress on established goals. The patient had set goals to keep food records, take medications, and have an eye exam by the end of the month. The patient can read back meals for 3 days and reports using a new phone app to remind the patient to take medications. The patient has not yet had an eye exam. Which statement is true about this patient's efforts in reducing risks?

    A. The patient is meeting goals for reducing risks
    B. The patient has not met the goals for reducing risks
    C. The patient needs to make a goal for reducing risks
    D. There is not enough information to evaluate

15. An 11-year-old patient with type 1 diabetes can successfully identify carbohydrates and describe their effects. What is the best new learning goal to continue ongoing plans for advancing the patient's diabetes knowledge and skills?

    A. Altering food intake based on glucose levels
    B. Creating a balanced meal plan in diabetes
    C. Adjusting insulin doses based on meal intake
    D. Identifying appropriate food when eating out

16. A patient with type 2 diabetes is being discharged from the hospital after treatment for a diabetes-related wound infection. The diabetes educator wants to assess the patient's knowledge before discharging them. What is an appropriate topic for discussion?

    A. Proper and consistent nutrition habits
    B. Complications of diabetes
    C. Psychosocial factors in managing diabetes
    D. Review of the patient's home glucose log

17. A patient with poorly controlled diabetes and a recent hip fracture is being discharged. Discharge needs include self-monitoring equipment, outpatient diabetes education, prescriptions, and home healthcare for physical therapy. The patient is not covered by Medicare Part D. Which of the following will be a concern for coverage?

    A. Home health
    B. Glucose meter and strips
    C. Prescriptions
    D. Further education

18. An adult patient with type 1 diabetes has an insulin correction factor of 1:30 and a carb-to-insulin ratio of 1:10. Their glucose before a 60-g meal is 190 with a premeal glucose goal of 100. How many units of insulin should they take?

    A. 3
    B. 6
    C. 9
    D. 12

19. An adult patient with a stated history of type 2 diabetes presents with weight loss, uncontrolled glucose, and a history of ketosis. The patient states that they are compliant with oral medications but the medications just are not working. What is the most probable explanation for the patient's condition?

   A. The patient has latent autoimmune diabetes in adults (LADA) and should begin insulin therapy
   B. The patient has maturity-onset diabetes of the young (MODY) and should begin insulin therapy
   C. The patient has LADA and should increase oral therapy
   D. The patient has MODY and should increase oral therapy

20. An older adult patient with type 2 diabetes wants to improve their exercise habits. The patient is not confident about being able to exercise the way their doctor wants because of advanced arthritis. Further discussion reveals that the patient demonstrates good knowledge of the benefits of exercise but has limited understanding of safe options. Which instructional method is most beneficial for this patient?

   A. Review two short videos on exercise options for seniors
   B. Provide a handout with listings of local senior gyms
   C. Discuss exercise shoe options to maintain foot safety
   D. Demonstrate safe chair exercises for the patient to do

21. An adult patient with newly diagnosed type 2 diabetes complains of pain when they prick their finger to test their blood glucose. The pain is causing them to not want to check their blood glucose levels. What could be a reason for this problem?

   A. They may be pricking the middle of their fingertip
   B. They may be using too small of a lancet gauge
   C. They may not be milking their fingers
   D. They may be dehydrated

22. A 15-year-old patient with type 1 diabetes needs instruction on carbohydrate counting and carbohydrate choices. To provide an example of carb counting, the patient is asked to write down what they ate the night before. They write: 1 cup of pasta, meat sauce, salad, one small piece of garlic bread, a ½ cup yogurt with ½ cup berries, and a diet soda. How many total carbohydrates were consumed?

   A. Two
   B. Four
   C. Six
   D. Eight

23. An adult patient has a history of type 1 diabetes. They would like to exercise more but are unsure what would be safe. They report a history of gastroparesis and heat intolerance. Their healthcare team suspects autonomic neuropathy. What is the appropriate response?

    A. Educate them on the risk of hypertension after vigorous activity
    B. Suggest recumbent cycling as a potential safe exercise
    C. Recommend proper timing of rapid-acting insulin
    D. Encourage warmer environments such as a hot yoga studio

24. An older adult patient with type 2 diabetes states that they have successfully completed some group diabetes classes. At follow-up, however, they cannot identify carbohydrate foods or evaluate a food label for carbohydrate content. The patient says they want to change habits but feels overwhelmed by not knowing what to eat. What can the diabetes educator determine from this patient's situation?

    A. The teaching was ineffective during the class, and the patient has not met learning objectives
    B. The teaching was ineffective for the patient's learning needs, and they need a new learning plan
    C. There is progress toward behavioral goals because the patient is willing to make diet changes
    D. There is progress toward learning goals because the patient successfully completed the class

25. An older adult patient has had type 2 diabetes for more than 6 years but reports that they never really learned about their medications and often skip them because they are afraid of the adverse effects. A review shows they were prescribed metformin and glyburide. What is an appropriate intermediate outcome to measure when educating this patient?

    A. Understanding medication side effects
    B. Measuring reduction in A1C
    C. Adhering to taking medications
    D. Tracking improvement in quality of life

26. An adult patient has a goal to decrease soft drink intake to reduce daily glucose levels. The patient was not aware that soft drinks were high in sugar and is not sure what alternatives to try. The patient is provided handouts, label-reading examples, and a list of alternatives to sugared beverages. What is the best way to evaluate meeting the learning goals for that session?

    A. Ask the patient to calculate carbohydrates from a beverage label
    B. Have the patient teach back negative effects of sugared beverages
    C. Assess the patient's drink choices at a 2-week follow-up visit
    D. Review glucose logs and evaluate changes in postmeal glucose

27. A 37-year-old patient with long-standing type 1 diabetes has a history of gastroparesis. A physical exam reveals trace edema, and the patient tests positive for orthostatic hypotension. Which advice should this patient receive?

    A. "Monitor your glucose frequently to check for hypoglycemia."
    B. "Wear proper shoes to protect your feet."
    C. "Most of your symptoms will resolve on their own."
    D. "Reorganize your home in such a way to prevent falls."

28. Glucose records for a patient with type 2 diabetes demonstrate a pattern. Their blood glucose was high at the same time of day on 2 nonconsecutive days during 1 week. Which is an appropriate plan of action?

    A. Recommend that the patient adjust their activity at that time of day
    B. Look for three or more consistent patterns
    C. Educate on the patient on foods that cause high blood glucose
    D. Advise the patient to increase their insulin by 10 units

29. The parents of an 8-year-old patient newly diagnosed with type 1 diabetes mention their concerns with their child's irregular bowel habits and abdominal pain. For what condition should the child be tested?

    A. Addison's disease
    B. Graves' disease
    C. Celiac disease
    D. Crohn's disease

30. A young adult patient with type 2 diabetes is frustrated that they have been unable to quit drinking soda despite their desire to change and reduce their soda intake. Which statement is an appropriate response using motivational interviewing?

    A. "What makes this change important to you?"
    B. "What is the risk of drinking soda?"
    C. "How does work or home affect your soda drinking?"
    D. "How does not meeting your goals make you feel?"

31. A patient taking insulin informs the diabetes educator that they consume large quantities of meat because it does not contain carbohydrate and so it should not impact their blood glucose. What is the educator's best response?

    A. "Meat won't impact your blood glucose, but the fat is still bad for your heart."
    B. "Large amounts of meat or fat can make your blood glucose higher, and you may need more insulin."
    C. "The protein in meat will actually make your blood glucose lower, so you'll need less insulin."
    D. "That's what makes low-carb diets so perfect for individuals with diabetes."

32. A patient who is under a great deal of financial strain states that they have been checking their blood glucose once a day at random times for the past 3 months, so they have used only 90 strips. What is the best response from the educator?

    A. "That's an economical way of doing things and should give us enough information to make adjustments."
    B. "It's very important that you test your glucose at least three times a day."
    C. "I would prefer that you test your glucose fasting and after meals on 2 days of the week."
    D. "Are there other areas of your budget you could cut back on? Nothing is more important than your health."

33. A 75-year-old patient with type 2 diabetes is being assessed for potential needs after several hospitalizations. They insist they can care for themself and are not ready to move into an assisted living facility. What would be an appropriate question to ask regarding their ability to perform activities of daily living?

    A. "Do you have trouble reading the paper or hearing the TV?"
    B. "How much help do you need with cooking?"
    C. "Are you able to walk without becoming short of breath?"
    D. "How often have you fallen in the last month?"

34. An 18-year-old female college student who has had type 1 diabetes for 5 years suddenly has unexplained elevations in her A1C and has been hospitalized with diabetic ketoacidosis three times in 3 months. Upon assessment, she states that she has kept the same medication regimen and denies changes in her activities. What would be an appropriate consideration?

    A. She should be assessed for diabetic distress
    B. She may need to be assessed for disordered eating behaviors
    C. She may need group counseling for adjustment disorder
    D. She needs counseling on the benefits of continuous glucose monitors

35. A patient reports that they regularly skip breakfast because they believe that it causes their blood glucose to be higher the rest of the day. What is the best response?

    A. "That is correct, so if you can skip it without becoming hypoglycemic, you should."
    B. "Breakfast may help glucose control by adding consistency to your meal plan."
    C. "It's fine to eat breakfast, but make sure it is almost all protein."
    D. "If you're exercising in the morning, it's better to do it on an empty stomach so that you'll burn more fat."

36. An adult patient newly diagnosed with type 2 diabetes states that they have always wanted to try a vegetarian diet but now believe that it is not a good idea for them because it would consist of too much carbohydrate. What is the best response?

    A. "Vegetarian diets are more successful than other diets."
    B. "It is really calorie restriction that helps improve glycemic control."
    C. "Have you looked into the DASH (Dietary Approaches to Stop Hypertension) diet, which may be more helpful?"
    D. "Have you ever considered trying more gluten-free foods?"

37. A patient with a 10-year history of type 2 diabetes and hypertension presents to the clinic for a routine exam. Urinalysis results include albuminuria of 230 mg/24 hr. What is the most appropriate education focus for this patient?

    A. They need to reduce sodium in their diet
    B. They need to reduce potassium in their diet
    C. They need to reduce protein in their diet
    D. They do not need to make any changes

38. A patient who plans to eat 45 g of carbohydrate at dinner says that their blood glucose has been running high after the evening meal. The patient states that they have been eating a lot of crab cakes but use only one slice of bread per two crab cakes. The patient eats two crab cakes, a cup of broccoli or cauliflower, and a cup of melon for dinner. Which question will best determine why the patient's blood glucose has been running high?

    A. "Are you using real crabmeat or imitation crab?"
    B. "What type of melon are you eating?"
    C. "Are you putting margarine on your vegetables?"
    D. "Do you put tartar sauce on your crab cakes?"

39. While providing a medication and supplement history, a patient states that they are taking several high-dose cinnamon supplements every day and using cinnamon often with meals. When asked about the purpose of the supplement, they reply, "I hear it is good to lower blood sugar. Since it is all natural, it can't be bad." What is the best response?

    A. "You're right, cinnamon is safe for you to use."
    B. "Large amounts of cinnamon are possibly toxic to the liver."
    C. "Large amounts of cinnamon might cause cancer."
    D. "Large amounts of cinnamon can be damaging to the kidneys."

40. A patient with type 2 diabetes has been making lifestyle changes. They state that they are trying to eat as little fat as possible in order to lose weight. What would be the best response?

    A. "Maintaining a low-fat diet is a good way to lose weight."
    B. "Focusing on the types of fat rather than reducing all fat can be more beneficial."
    C. "Keep your fat intake at about 15% to 20% of your calories."
    D. "Supplements are also beneficial when reducing fat in your diet."

41. A patient reports that they ate three eggs, three pieces of whole wheat toast with butter, a large banana, and ½ cup of orange juice for breakfast because they knew that their lunch was going to be later than usual. How many carbohydrate choices did they eat at breakfast?

    A. Three
    B. Four
    C. Five
    D. Six

42. Which phrase best describes the cause of maturity-onset diabetes of the young?

    A. A genetic defect affecting beta cell function
    B. An autoimmune destruction of the beta cells
    C. An insulin resistance
    D. A hormonal disorder affecting glucose metabolism

43. A patient is able to adjust their insulin based on a ratio of carbohydrate consumed to doses of rapid-acting insulin. Their current carbohydrate-to-insulin ratio is 12:1. They eat a 60-g carbohydrate lunch. How many insulin units would they bolus for their meal?

    A. 12
    B. 24
    C. 48
    D. 72

44. During their initial assessment, the patient tells the educator that they will be observing Ramadan the following month and thus will be fasting from dawn until sunset every day for 30 days. Which instruction is most important for the educator to provide?

    A. "Aim to maintain portion control when you do have meals."
    B. "You may need to exercise more to help with glucose control."
    C. "Be sure to continue to take your oral medications as instructed."
    D. "Check your glucose after you eat to avoid hyperglycemia."

45. An older adult patient is tearful and tells the diabetes educator that they have gained 35 lb in the past 5 years. The patient insists that they do not eat any processed foods or sweets. They take metformin and insulin and have no other health concerns that could explain the weight gain. They often skip meals entirely and have at least one or two episodes of hypoglycemia each week. What should the educator's next question be?

    A. "What dosage of metformin are you on?"
    B. "Do you think that you might be depressed?"
    C. "What would you like to weigh?"
    D. "How are you correcting your hypoglycemia?"

46. An adult patient newly diagnosed with diabetes asks about medications that will work immediately to lower blood glucose. Which medication will have an immediate effect?

    A. Januvia
    B. Metformin
    C. Rosiglitazone
    D. Acarbose

47. A patient with a continuous glucose monitor experienced a blood glucose of 50. To treat the low glucose level, they took three glucose tablets containing 20 g of carbohydrate. They rechecked 15 minutes later and their monitor showed that their glucose was still low, so they drank 1/3 cup of grape juice. About 30 minutes later, their glucose was too high. Which statement best explains this patient's high glucose level?

    A. They should have had apple juice instead of grape juice
    B. They needed to use more glucose tablets at the outset
    C. They should have waited half an hour before rechecking the monitor
    D. They should have used a finger-stick reading rather than the continuous monitor

48. A patient has been eating several servings of cookies sweetened with sugar alcohol every day because they are "free foods" and do not count as carbohydrate. What should the educator tell the patient about this practice?

    A. Sugar alcohols are nonnutritive, so although they reduce the calories in a food, the food is not a "free food"

    B. Sugar alcohols are lower in calories because they are poorly absorbed and can cause digestive distress

    C. As long as the product is labeled "sugar-free," it is a free food and does not need to be counted

    D. Sugar alcohols come from fruits and berries, so they should be counted as a serving of fruit

49. A young adult patient has well-controlled insulin-dependent diabetes. The patient will be traveling to a different time zone for a 2-week vacation next month. What would be an appropriate suggestion?

    A. Stay on schedule injecting insulin in your home time zone

    B. Have a snack plan to avoid low blood sugars

    C. Test glucose levels when necessary to avoid stress

    D. Have medications sent ahead to avoid flight issues

50. A patient with type 2 diabetes, hypertension, and high cholesterol provides laboratory results for review. The lab results are: glucose 99 mg/dL, glomerular filtration rate 40, total cholesterol 179 mg/dL, low-density lipoprotein 62 mg/dL, and triglycerides 135 mg/dL. What is of greatest concern for this patient after reviewing the labs?

    A. The patient is hypoglycemic and needs to reduce medications

    B. The patient has not been taking their cholesterol medication

    C. The patient may need medication dose changes for chronic kidney disease

    D. There are no concerns; the lab results are normal

51. A patient with type 2 diabetes has a 15-year smoking history. The patient reports having heard that heard e-cigarettes could help with quitting. What advice should be given?

    A. E-cigarettes are a healthier alternative but may not help with quitting

    B. E-cigarettes have not been shown to be an effective way to quit

    C. E-cigarettes are worse than smoking for the heart and lungs

    D. E-cigarettes could be a good alternative to a nicotine patch

52. A patient who has had diabetes for more than 20 years had localized lipo-hypertrophy during a recent physical assessment. What should the diabetes educator be sure to talk to the patient about?

   A. Not reusing needles

   B. Avoiding intramuscular injection

   C. Rotating insulin injection sites

   D. Changing needle size

53. A patient presents with complaints of poor appetite, weakness, trouble concentrating, and fluid retention. What condition should the diabetes educator suspect in this patient?

   A. Kidney disease

   B. Liver disease

   C. Congestive heart failure

   D. Stroke

54. A patient with well-controlled diabetes plans to take a road trip and will be in the car for 10 to 12 hours each way. The patient has been taking insulin for 5 years. How often should the patient test their blood glucose while on the road?

   A. Only if they have symptoms of hypoglycemia

   B. Before driving and at regular intervals

   C. Every 6 hours

   D. They should not drive for long periods of time

55. A patient brings their most recent lipid panel results to a checkup with the diabetes educator. Their results are cholesterol 190, high-density lipoprotein (HDL) 60, low-density lipoprotein (LDL) 90, and triglycerides 210. Which note does the educator write in the patient's file about their results?

   A. Their cholesterol is too high, and their HDL is too low

   B. Their LDL is too high, and their HDL is too low

   C. Their triglycerides are too high, and everything else is normal

   D. Their LDL and triglycerides are both too high

56. A patient at 28 weeks of gestation takes a one-step method glucose tolerance test with the following results: 70 mg/dL fasting; 175 mg/dL at 1 hour; 163 mg/dL at 2 hours. What do these results indicate?

    A. Normal results for a pregnant patient
    B. A high 1-hour level
    C. A high 2-hour level
    D. A need for further testing

57. A patient with a long history of type 2 diabetes reports sudden onset of weakness and excruciating pain in the muscles of the thigh, hip, and buttocks. The patient is most likely describing which condition?

    A. Diabetic amyotrophy
    B. Autonomic neuropathy
    C. Chronic inflammatory demyelinating polyneuropathy
    D. Charcot–Marie–Tooth disease

58. Which mineral is typically administered along with insulin when a person is hospitalized with diabetic ketoacidosis?

    A. Sodium
    B. Chloride
    C. Potassium
    D. Phosphorus

59. A patient who suffered multiple bone fractures and contusions in a car accident is being discharged home with pain medication as needed. The patient is on pramlintide. What advice should the educator give the patient regarding medications?

    A. Stop taking pramlintide and start on acarbose while taking pain medications
    B. The pain medication and pramlintide can be taken at the same time without interaction
    C. The pain medication should not be taken within 2 hours of pramlintide
    D. The dosage of pramlintide will need to be increased while taking pain medication

60. A patient with poorly controlled diabetes has a gastric emptying test showing 15% after 4 hours of food intake. What food recommendation would be appropriate?

    A. High-fiber diet
    B. Low-fat diet
    C. Gluten-free diet
    D. Lactose-free diet

61. A 78-year-old patient with a long history of type 2 diabetes describes an incident of sudden pain and inability to move the shoulder. The patient reports that the pain then went away. What is the most likely explanation for this episode?

    A. Charcot joint
    B. Entrapment syndrome
    C. Diabetic amyotrophy
    D. Mononeuropathy

62. Which patient statement should alert the educator to consider recommending the involvement of a mental health professional?

    A. "I feel tired at times but not all of the time."
    B. "I have no appetite and I've lost 10 lb this month."
    C. "I've been trying to work on my crafts several times a week."
    D. "At least I think things will get better next month."

63. An adult patient is newly diagnosed with diabetes. The diabetes educator notices that the patient often interrupts during conversations, asks for more details, and shares specific problems. What would be the most useful strategy in further educating the patient?

    A. Providing a video on living with diabetes
    B. Offering a motivational book on coping
    C. Using a conversation map about taking medications
    D. Setting up food models when teaching meal planning

64. A young adult patient with type 1 diabetes voices frustration because they are a violin player and their fingertips get sore from testing frequently. The patient has purchased an alternate site meter and asks whether it can be used for all readings. What is the educator's most appropriate response?

    A. "It can be accurate, but readings will be lower than if you use your fingertips."
    B. "It is good as an emergency backup, such as when traveling."
    C. "It can serve as another meter when you want to compare readings."
    D. "Readings will not reflect any rapid changes in glucose levels."

65. A patient wants to modify their diet to benefit their heart and blood pressure. The patient asks the diabetes educator to explain the major difference between the Mediterranean diet and the DASH (Dietary Approaches to Stop Hypertension) diet. Which statement is the educator's best response?

    A. The Mediterranean diet is more plant-based than the DASH diet
    B. The DASH diet limits dairy foods
    C. The Mediterranean diet allows meat
    D. The DASH diet emphasizes sodium restriction

66. A patient recently lost their spouse and is now in the denial stage of grief. What is the best approach for the educator to take for providing diabetes education during this time?

    A. Try to distract the patient so they can focus on the diabetes education
    B. Be willing to listen and focus on basic skills and concepts
    C. Try to get the patient to talk about their feelings in a group education setting
    D. Recommend an antidepressant to the patient

67. The nutrition facts label on a package of cookies states that there are 22 g of carbohydrate in one serving. How many carbohydrate choices are in two servings of the cookies?

    A. One
    B. Two
    C. Three
    D. Four

68. A 35-year-old patient with a history of gestational diabetes has a height of 5'4" and weighed 245 lb before pregnancy. They are starting their third trimester and weigh 252 lb. What advice can be given regarding the weight gain?

    A. The patient is gaining an appropriate amount of weight
    B. The patient should aim to gain another pound a week
    C. The patient is not gaining enough weight
    D. The patient needs to aim to gain an additional 15 lb

69. A patient with type 2 diabetes, hypertension, and albuminuria states that they do not understand why their doctor told them an angiotensin-converting enzyme (ACE) inhibitor or angiotensin receptor blocker (ARB) are the best options for them. What is the diabetes educator's best response to this question?

    A. Other medications raise blood glucose
    B. Other medications increase the risk of infection
    C. ACE inhibitors and ARBs reduce the risk of progressive kidney disease
    D. ACE inhibitors and ARBs promote weight loss

70. The parents of a 16-year-old patient who was diagnosed with type 1 diabetes at age 4 express a desire to help but also want the patient to be independent. They ask what they can do to help while respecting the patient's boundaries. Which statement is the educator's best response?

    A. "Be reassuring, and provide positive reinforcement."
    B. "Set behavioral limits, but expect a lack of adherence."
    C. "Assist in regular glucose monitoring."
    D. "Ask your child what is helpful for you to do."

71. An adult patient is being educated about glucose monitoring. They have newly diagnosed diabetes but are not taking medication for the diabetes. When questioned about their eating habits, they state that their largest meal is often at dinner. What structured testing plan would be most helpful?

    A. Three-point profile
    B. Staggered profile
    C. Meal-based profile
    D. Five-point profile

72. A young adult patient with type 1 diabetes describes weight loss and increased appetite, heat intolerance, heart palpitations, muscle weakness, and irregular menstrual periods. The patient's blood glucose readings, which are generally on target, have become irregular and sporadic. To which specialist should the diabetes educator consider referring the patient?

    A. Endocrinologist for symptoms of Graves' disease
    B. Psychiatrist for symptoms of an eating disorder
    C. Rheumatologist for symptoms of multiple sclerosis
    D. Nephrologist for symptoms of kidney failure

73. Which hormone reduces the muscle uptake of glucose during exercise?

    A. Growth hormone
    B. Cortisol
    C. Norepinephrine
    D. Glucagon

74. An older adult patient has type 2 diabetes. At a prior visit, the patient was educated about food labels, was instructed to limit carbohydrates to 45 to 60 g per meal, and was given written instructions. Upon return, the patient reports that their glucose levels are even higher, and they are adamant that they have been measuring their carbohydrates appropriately. What skill is this patient most likely lacking?

    A. Literacy
    B. Numeracy
    C. Document literacy
    D. Prose literacy

75. The director of a diabetes education program states that development of behavioral objectives must be used for evaluation of program outcomes. Which statement is the most appropriate example of a behavioral objective?

    A. The participant will demonstrate the ability to safely and accurately monitor their blood glucose
    B. The participant will know what diabetes is
    C. The participant will believe that they can achieve lifestyle modifications to control their diabetes
    D. The participant will understand which diabetes supplies are usually covered by insurance

76. A review of the clinic schedule shows that a patient scheduled for the afternoon is hearing impaired. What is the most appropriate way to prepare for working with this patient?

    A. Schedule interpreter services to be available for the session
    B. Plan to show a video with sign language on living with diabetes
    C. Set up a white board to use for instruction
    D. Ensure a family member will be present to assist in education

77. A 54-year-old patient with type 2 diabetes diagnosed 2 years ago has an A1C of 10.5% and blood pressure of 154/92 mmHg. The patient is referred for diabetes education after a hospitalization related to uncontrolled diabetes mellitus and blood pressure. The patient reports that they got tired of taking their medications because they felt sicker when taking them and believed they were not working. They state that they have cut back on sodas and started to eat healthier, take vitamins, and walk every day. They have a goal to be a great-grandparent. What is an appropriate action for the diabetes educator?

    A. Review information on target goals and the safety of medications
    B. Provide encouragement to achieve the goal of becoming a
       great-grandparent
    C. Document concerns for noncompliance and refer the patient to a
       cardiologist
    D. Reinforce further lifestyle interventions and encourage supplements

78. A patient presents to the primary care clinic with malaise, fatigue, frequent urination, thirst, and dizziness. Test results show glucose of 230 and an A1C of 15.5%. Which is an appropriate initial therapy for this patient?

    A. Metformin and basal insulin
    B. Basal bolus
    C. Metformin and lifestyle changes
    D. Basal insulin and glucagon-like peptide-1 (GLP-1) receptor

79. A patient reports not checking glucose as often as they should and cites a busy open-office workplace where it is inconvenient to self-test. What would be an appropriate follow-up solution?

    A. Set up reminder aids
    B. Review necessary skills
    C. Suggest private spaces
    D. Acknowledge feelings

80. An A1C test may be performed to diagnose diabetes if a patient has a body mass index (BMI) of 28 and the patient:

   A. Is in the third trimester of pregnancy
   B. Has had a recent blood transfusion
   C. Has polycystic ovary syndrome
   D. Is on erythropoietin therapy

81. A patient just started checking blood pressure at home but is unsure if they are doing it correctly. What is appropriate advice?

   A. Check the blood pressure after exercising to compare it with resting blood pressure
   B. Purchase a cuff that fits snugly to be sure it fits around the arm
   C. Measure the pressure several times 1 minute apart, and record the results
   D. Check the blood pressure at a local pharmacy to compare readings

82. When working with a patient diagnosed with type 2 diabetes and metabolic stress syndrome on developing a self-management plan, the educator would explain that a primary factor leading to hyperglycemia in this patient is:

   A. Decrease in hepatic glucose production that is needed to regulate blood glucose
   B. Increase in peripheral muscle uptake of glucose that prevents insulin from circulating in the body
   C. Decrease in production of incretin hormones that promote insulin production after eating
   D. Decrease in kidney reabsorption of glucose causing the body to be depleted of needed blood sugar

83. An older adult patient presents with mild abdominal pain, nausea, and vomiting for the past several days. Blood glucose levels are above 800 mg/dL. The patient is afebrile, and the breath is normal. Which step would be performed first?

   A. Contact the provider for an order to initiate insulin therapy
   B. Refer to the emergency department to begin intravenous fluid replacement
   C. Obtain an A1C level and have the patient wait while labs are processed
   D. Order testing for zinc transporter antibodies

84. The manager of a diabetes program is asked about the effectiveness of the program in changing behaviors. A review of a sample of patient charts reveals that the data accumulated are insufficient. What is an appropriate next step?

    A. Initiate calls to reach patients in 3 months for follow-up
    B. Revise the education documentation to include behaviors
    C. Obtain charts to review documentation of chosen behavior data
    D. Conduct an in-service session for staff on documenting outcomes

85. A patient with a previous diagnosis of gestational diabetes has an abnormal oral glucose tolerance test (OGTT) at 12 weeks of pregnancy. The diabetes educator advises that after delivery the patient's blood glucose levels will most likely:

    A. Return to normal within 24 to 48 hours
    B. Increase suddenly and need to be monitored in the hospital
    C. Remain elevated and require the same therapy that was used in pregnancy
    D. Remain elevated and require further monitoring to determine therapy

86. A 16-year-old patient with type 1 diabetes brings in their blood glucose log for review. The patient takes 30 units of long-acting insulin before bed and rapid-acting insulin based on a carbohydrate ratio of 1 to 10 and a correction factor of 1:50. The patient's blood glucose log recordings are:
    Day 1: Fasting: 66; Prelunch: 178; Predinner: 137; Bedtime: 143

    Day 2: Fasting: 83; Prelunch: 128; Predinner: 120; Bedtime: 110

    Day 3: Fasting: 69; Prelunch: 139; Predinner: 107; Bedtime: 105

    What change in the plan should be implemented?

    A. Decrease the dose of long-acting insulin to 24 units before bed
    B. Decrease the dose of long-acting insulin to 20 units before bed
    C. Split the dose of long-acting insulin into 15 units in the morning and 15 units before bed
    D. Change the carbohydrate ratio to 1 to 8

87. A 16-year-old patient on insulin pump therapy presents to the hospital in diabetic ketoacidosis. The patient does not have a continuous glucose monitor due to adverse reactions to adhesives in the past. During assessment, it is noted that the patient has lost 8 lb (3.6 kg) in 2 weeks, and the patient confides that they have been keeping their pump confined to a backpack at school (allowing the basal insulin to drain into a tissue). The patient admits to administering a bolus prior to arrival home so their parents won't be suspicious. In prioritizing the patient's plan of care, what area will be the focus of intervention?

   A. Instruct the patient to maintain a blood sugar level between 80 and 130 preprandial and <180 postprandial
   B. Provide interventions that will achieve blood glucose level normalization immediately
   C. Discuss ways the patient can keep the pump off temporarily but still achieve blood sugar goals
   D. Work with the patient to set realistic blood sugar goals initially post discharge

88. When teaching a patient about meal planning and blood glucose control, which statement best fits the recommended approach?

   A. Eating meals only when hungry is an important part of diabetes management
   B. Learn how to quantify carbohydrate intake to match mealtime insulin doses
   C. Insulin should be taken postprandial based on total grams of carbohydrate consumed in the meal
   D. Carbohydrate consumption can be unlimited provided the carbohydrates are "covered" by the appropriate dose of insulin

89. Which clinical finding indicates that it is appropriate to begin screening a patient for prediabetes?

   A. Body mass index (BMI) 22 kg/m²
   B. Triglycerides 200 mg/dL
   C. Age 35 years
   D. Blood pressure (BP) 127/86 mmHg

90. A 17-year-old patient with type 1 diabetes complains of dizziness and nausea every evening after sports practice. The patient's blood glucose levels prior to exercise range from 100 to 130 mg/dL. What will the diabetes educator recommend to this patient?

    A. Lower basal insulin rate by 60% to compensate for exertion
    B. Consume 30 to 60 g of carbohydrates prior to practice
    C. Discontinue all strenuous athletic activities
    D. Skip practice if blood glucose level is not between 126 and 180 mg/dL

91. A patient with uncontrolled type 2 diabetes has repeatedly canceled their education sessions. The patient lives in a rural area and cites various reasons for canceling, including transportation issues and inclement weather. The patient expresses interest in the appointment and continues to reschedule. What action will the educator take to help ensure the patient's needs are met?

    A. Inform the primary care provider that the patient is noncompliant
    B. Postpone any scheduled visits
    C. Offer the option of a telemedicine visit
    D. Send the patient a letter detailing the benefits of the education service

92. The educator is discussing medication management with a patient with type 2 diabetes who was started on low-dose metformin 6 months earlier. Since that time, the patient has not been able to reach the desired glycemic targets. To avoid therapeutic inertia, the educator will discuss which next step with the patient?

    A. Continuing the current regimen
    B. Intensifying the medication regimen
    C. Following up in 3 months to reassess
    D. Allowing the patient more time to reach the targets

93. How will the educator initiate a conversation when problem-solving with a teenage patient struggling with type 1 diabetes management and their family?

    A. Have the patient and the family discuss each issue that they are having with the patient's diabetes management
    B. Have the family members use language such as, "I feel hurt because of the way you handle your diabetes."
    C. Begin by selecting one problem to be discussed and have everyone state the problem clearly, using "I" statements
    D. Identify the oldest family member as the primary communicator in the discussion

94. The most frequent cause of hyperglycemia in clinical practice is:

    A. Corticosteroid drug use
    B. Septic infection
    C. Excessive carbohydrate intake
    D. Inadequate insulin dosing

95. An adult patient with type 2 diabetes is being seen after a recent hospitaliza-
    tion. The patient was hospitalized for non-diabetes-related issues and was on
    the general medical floor. The patient reports being on subcutaneous insu-
    lin during hospitalization with a glycemic target of 80 to 130 mg/dL, which
    resulted in several hypoglycemic episodes. What action will the educator
    take?

    A. Explain to the patient that each hospital floor has different goals
    B. Explain to the patient that this is an appropriate goal for the current
       hospitalization
    C. Apologize to the patient and explain there is nothing the educator can do
       since this occurred in the hospital
    D. Set up an education session for general medicine floor providers and
       nurses

96. A patient with generally well-controlled diabetes calls the clinic complaining
    of hypoglycemia over the last week. The patient is currently taking metformin
    (Glucophage) and simvastatin (Zocor). Upon further discussion, a sprained
    ankle is reported, and the patient admits taking acetylsalicylic acid (aspirin)
    "around the clock" with little monitoring due to a busy work schedule. What
    is the most appropriate educational topic at this time?

    A. Information on drug interactions between simvastatin (Zocor) and acetyl-
       salicylic acid (aspirin)
    B. Importance of prioritizing health and managing stress levels
    C. Effect of trauma and injury on blood glucose levels
    D. Correlation of high doses of acetylsalicylic acid (aspirin) to hypoglycemia

97. An older adult patient with type 2 diabetes is taking 100 units of insulin glargine (Lantus) and 500 mg twice daily of metformin. Fasting blood glucose readings have been 80 to 100 mg/dL with A1C of 7.6%. The estimated glomerular filtration rate (eGFR) has decreased from 55 mL/min/1.73 m^2 to 40 mL/min/1.73 m^2. Based on the current status, which change to the patient's medication regimen is most likely to be recommended?

    A. Make no changes at this time
    B. Increase metformin to 1,000 mg twice daily
    C. Add empagliflozin (Jardiance)
    D. Increase insulin glargine (Lantus) to 115 units

98. Following a provider's assessment for cardiovascular disease and permission to prescribe an exercise plan, what initial strategy would be appropriate?

    A. Advise the patient to start out doing at least 150 minutes of exercise every week and build up from there
    B. Discuss the patient's physical abilities and interests and help them set realistic goals following this assessment
    C. Recommend 2 days a week of resistance training and 150 minutes of cardiovascular exercise throughout the week
    D. Facilitate beginning high-intensity interval training 3 days a week for 30 minutes for optimal blood sugar levels

99. A patient with well-controlled type 2 diabetes reports recently becoming pregnant. After confirming normal blood glucose readings on the current insulin lispro (Humalog), what will the nurse advise?

    A. Switch to glargine (Lantus) because long-acting insulin is safer during pregnancy
    B. Advise patient to continue the current plan as long as normal blood glucose levels are maintained
    C. Discontinue insulin and switch to oral medications because insulin crosses the placenta
    D. Initiate therapy using an insulin pump

100. A young adult patient is referred to the clinic. The patient denies symptoms of hyperglycemia or complications of diabetes. A1C is 9.1% with a fasting blood glucose of 185. The patient's past medical history is unremarkable. Urine ketones are negative, fasting C-peptide is 0.9 (0.8–3.85), and insulin antibody is <0.4 units/mL (0–1). The patient's father was diagnosed with diabetes at age 18 years, takes metformin, and has reported good control without complications. The patient is diagnosed with diabetes, but further diagnostic tests are required to ascertain diabetes type. Which of the following tests would the diabetes educator request to be ordered?

   A. Repeat postprandial glucose, thyroid-stimulating hormone (TSH), anti-thyroid antibodies, and glutamic acid decarboxylase (GAD) antibodies
   B. Nonfasting C-peptide level, hemoglobin, TSH, and antithyroid antibodies
   C. Another A1C and postprandial glucose
   D. GAD antibodies, anti-islet cell antibodies, fasting insulin, nonfasting C-peptide levels, TSH, and antithyroid antibodies

101. When the A1C and the glucose log do not match, what user factor should be evaluated as the most likely reason for the mismatch?

   A. Time the glucose level was taken
   B. Site where the specimen was taken
   C. Glucose level at the time of testing
   D. Brand of glucose testing strips that were used

102. When educating a patient about special circumstances that require additional glucose records, what circumstance would be included?

   A. Patient illness
   B. Temperature shifts
   C. Patient's new job
   D. Weather changes

103. Hyperosmolar hyperglycemic syndrome (HHS) is most likely to be seen in a patient who:

   A. Drinks 2 L of water per day
   B. Has a urinary tract infection with or without symptoms
   C. Has eaten a meal with more than 80 g of carbohydrates
   D. Is a young adult

104. A 16-year-old patient has a recent diagnosis of type 1 diabetes and is experiencing depression. How can the diabetes educator demonstrate that an intervention for this patient was provided?

   A. Tell the patient that things will be fine and there is no reason to be depressed
   B. Describe how the educator's family member handles their diabetes to provide an example for the patient
   C. Refer patient to a psychologist, counselor, psychiatrist, or social worker
   D. Explain to the patient that their depression is likely hormonal and will improve as they age

105. Which of the following is included in the problem-solving guide to be used when setting goals with a patient with diabetes?

   A. Imagine an ideal scenario
   B. Come up with solutions on your own
   C. Identify the problem
   D. Set an action plan for a long-term goal

106. A patient who was screened for diabetes has the following laboratory results: fasting plasma glucose (FPG): 106; A1C: 6.5; repeat A1C: 6.7. What is the diagnosis for this patient?

   A. Prediabetes
   B. Abnormal glucose tolerance
   C. Euglycemia
   D. Diabetes

107. A patient is reluctant to test their glucose. Which of the following instructional methods is most likely to motivate them?

   A. Have the patient test glucose levels before and after eating foods they dislike
   B. Advise the patient to test when they feel well to see if it shows in glucose levels
   C. Negotiate a testing strategy that is based on what the patient is willing to do
   D. Have someone else do the patient's testing at home for a week

108. A patient with new-onset type 2 diabetes and uncontrolled hypertension is seen in the clinic. The provider places the patient on metformin, but no blood pressure medication has been ordered. What goal for the patient would be suggested by the educator?

    A. Instruct the patient in lifestyle changes and recommend that they return to the clinic in 1 month to have their blood pressure checked
    B. Instruct the patient in lifestyle changes and recommend that the provider start the patient on a medication for blood pressure
    C. Instruct the patient to monitor their blood pressure at home for 1 week and then return to the clinic for evaluation
    D. Instruct the patient in lifestyle changes and advise them to return to the clinic if they do not feel better in 2 weeks

109. When evaluating the cause of hypoglycemia, which factor should be included in the logging of glucose levels?

    A. Place testing was done
    B. Assistance patient received with testing
    C. Emotional condition of patient
    D. Timing of insulin use

110. All of the following are considered acute complications of diabetes except:

    A. Diabetes ketoacidosis (DKA)
    B. Hypoglycemia
    C. Hyperosmolar hyperglycemic syndrome (HHS)
    D. Peripheral neuropathy

111. A patient is diagnosed with prediabetes. What is the best resource for this patient?

    A. National Diabetes Prevention Program
    B. Living with Diabetes Educational Series
    C. American Heart Association
    D. U.S. Department of Agriculture

112. Which assessment question is the lowest priority for the patient with a new diagnosis of type 1 diabetes?

    A. What is your favorite way to learn?
    B. How far did you go in school?
    C. Would you describe yourself as forgetful?
    D. How optimistic are you about your diagnosis?

113. The patient's provider has prescribed regular insulin to be administered for meals. The patient's insurance plan covers rapid-acting insulin preparations. Based on the diabetes educator's recommendation, the provider changes the insulin order from regular to rapid acting. What best describes why the educator advocated for the change?

   A. Rapid-acting insulin has a faster absorption at 15 minutes, making it more conducive to improved glucose levels postprandial

   B. Regular insulin has an onset of 0.75 to 1 hour and can cause spikes in glucose postprandial if not taken before the meal

   C. Rapid-acting insulin takes 0.5 hour to onset, and regular insulin takes 0.5 to 1 hour for onset, making rapid insulin a better choice for meal planning

   D. Rapid-acting insulin is covered by the patient's insurance plan, so it makes sense financially to use rapid-acting insulin instead of regular insulin

114. When should questions and concerns identified by the patient be addressed during the educational process?

   A. At the end of the process once the basic information has already been provided

   B. During the assessment

   C. Once the diabetes educator and the patient have developed a rapport

   D. During the outcome evaluation

115. A teenage patient has uncontrolled diabetes. They rarely test their blood glucose levels. The patient's parents have a hands-off approach due to conflict with the teenager but are concerned about rising glucose levels and complications. The educator suspects miscarried helping. Which of the following methods is least beneficial in helping the patient's and parents' situation?

   A. Ask the parents and the patient who is responsible for certain aspects of the diabetes regimen

   B. Ask the patient how many minutes a day they spend tending to all of their diabetes care

   C. Ask the patient how many hours during the day the parents "nag" them about their diabetes

   D. Ask the parents to get more involved with the patient's glucose testing

116. A patient is new to insulin but is not eligible for a continuous glucose monitor due to insurance issues. The diabetes educator and the patient discuss ways to help the patient with tracking glucose and insulin dosing. The educator knows that the patient needs further education when they state:

    A. "I will write down my glucose levels and insulin dosing in a log book."
    B. "I can get a glucose monitor that can be downloaded in the doctor's office."
    C. "I can obtain a glucose meter that will transmit to my smart phone."
    D. "I will not worry because tracking my glucose and my insulin dosing is not important."

117. Which patient would be the least optimal candidate for insulin pump therapy? A patient who:

    A. Is planning for pregnancy
    B. Has frequent low blood glucose levels
    C. Does not use insulin-to-carbohydrate ratios
    D. Has an erratic schedule

118. When a diabetes educator is teaching a patient with diabetes, what is the least effective follow-up intervention?

    A. Telephone follow-up
    B. Video or internet-based program
    C. In-person shared medical appointment
    D. Virtual appointment with a registered dietitian nutritionist

119. A patient with type 1 diabetes states that they are burdened by calculating their insulin doses and keeping track of their insulin on board (IOB) to make treatment decisions. They also share that they do not want anything attached to their body. Which diabetes technology device would best match their needs and preferences?

    A. Implanted sensor
    B. Intermittent continuous glucose monitoring (CGM)
    C. Connected insulin pen
    D. Tubeless insulin pump therapy

120. Which pattern is optimal to educate a patient who requires premixed 70/30 neutral protamine hagedorn (NPH)/regular insulin?

   A. Onset (hours): <0.25; peak: dual; effective duration (hours): 10–16
   B. Onset (hours): <0.5–1; peak: dual; effective duration (hours): 10–16
   C. Onset (hours): <0.5; peak: dual; effective duration (hours): 20–24
   D. Onset (hours): <0.5; peak: dual; effective duration (hours): 10–12

121. Which basal to bolus strategy would the diabetes educator teach to the patient newly diagnosed with type 1 diabetes?

   A. Basal insulin accounts for 40% of the total daily insulin, and the bolus should account for 70% (divided into three doses for meals)
   B. Basal insulin accounts for 40% to 60% of the total daily insulin, and the bolus should account for the remaining percentage (divided into three doses for meals)
   C. Basal insulin accounts for 40% of the total daily insulin, and the bolus should account for 60% (divided into three doses for meals)
   D. Basal insulin accounts for 80% of the total daily insulin, and the bolus should account for 20% (divided into three doses for meals)

122. The patient is prescribed inhaled human insulin. On which insulin time frame should the patient receive education?

   A. Onset (hours): <0.25; peak: 2 (hours); effective duration (hours): 4
   B. Onset (hours): <0.25–0.5; peak: 0.25 (hours); effective duration (hours): 2
   C. Onset (hours): <0.01–0.05; peak: 0.12–0.15 (hours); effective duration (hours): 3
   D. Onset (hours): <0.25; peak: 1 (hours); effective duration (hours): 3

123. Which assessment question helps the patient with diabetes incorporate new behaviors to improve disease management?

   A. "Why do you choose to not check your blood glucose levels?"
   B. "Is checking your blood glucose levels difficult for you?"
   C. "Do you check your blood glucose levels when you're away from home?"
   D. "How important is checking your blood glucose levels to you?"

124. A patient with type 1 diabetes notices that when they correct for hyperglycemia before meals, their blood sugar remains elevated for 3 to 5 hours. What is the best explanation for the blood sugar elevation?

    A. The correction factor needs to be decreased
    B. 3 to 5 hours is a normal amount of time to see a blood sugar correction
    C. Hyperglycemia should be prevented rather than corrected
    D. The carbohydrate ratio is not strong enough

125. Oxidative stress would be triggered by an increase in postprandial glucose of more than:

    A. 50 mg/dL
    B. 20 mg/dL
    C. 80 mg/dL
    D. 100 mg/dL

126. When should adults newly diagnosed with type 1 diabetes be referred to ophthalmology for an initial dilated and comprehensive eye examination?

    A. At the time of their diagnosis
    B. 5 years after their diagnosis
    C. 2 years after their diagnosis if glycemia is well controlled
    D. 1 year after their diagnosis

127. Which age is most appropriate to begin transfer planning with patients transitioning from pediatric to adult care?

    A. 18 to 21 years
    B. 14 years
    C. 11 to 12 years
    D. 15 to 17 years

128. At which four critical times should healthcare team members evaluate the need for diabetes self-management education and support (DSMES) for their patients with diabetes?

    A. At diagnosis, annually, when the A1C is >9%, and when transitions in life and care occur

    B. 6 months after the patient has completed a diabetes self-management education (DSME) program, when the patient does not meet treatment targets, when insulin therapy is initiated, and when the patient requests DSMES

    C. At diagnosis, annually, when insulin therapy is initiated, and when complications of diabetes develop

    D. At diagnosis, annually and/or when the patient does not meet treatment targets, when factors develop that influence self-management, and when transitions in life and care occur

129. A patient with gestational diabetes is prescribed insulin. What is the most effective way to ensure insulin doses match the patient's insulin needs?

    A. Use guidelines based on weight and gestational age to determine insulin doses

    B. Teach the patient to make self-adjustments based on glucose data, food intake, and activity level

    C. Instruct the patient to keep a glucose log and bring it to their appointments

    D. Contact the patient to obtain glucose data and adjust doses in between visits

130. A patient with uncontrolled type 2 diabetes shares that they are not taking their prescribed medications due to fear of hypoglycemia and costs. Which two classes of medications should their provider prescribe?

    A. Biguanide and thiazolidinedione

    B. Second-generation sulfonylurea and thiazolidinedione

    C. Biguanide and long-acting insulin

    D. Biguanide and glucagon-like peptide 1 (GLP-1) receptor agonist

131. A patient sets a goal of walking 4 days a week for 30 minutes a day during their initial session with the diabetes educator. At the next follow-up appointment, the patient states that they have not started walking yet due to working long hours. Which would be an appropriate next intervention?

    A. Schedule the patient for a follow-up in 6 months to allow more time to achieve the goal

    B. Provide digital coaching to the patient

    C. Reassess the goal with the patient and consider possible revisions

    D. Ask the patient how they will feel after they achieve their goal

132. A patient on multiple daily injections of insulin brings their blood glucose log to the provider for review. The log shows a pattern of fasting blood sugars between 60 and 90, preprandial blood sugars between 150 and 180 before breakfast, and preprandial blood sugars between 110 and 130 before lunch and dinner. Which would be the most appropriate recommendation from the provider?

    A. Increase their mealtime insulin with breakfast and decrease their long-acting insulin
    B. Increase their mealtime insulin with lunch and decrease their long-acting insulin
    C. Decrease their long-acting insulin
    D. Have their breakfast earlier in the day

133. Increased insulin sensitivity post physical activity lasts approximately how many hours?

    A. 12
    B. 24
    C. 36
    D. 48

134. A patient recently diagnosed with type 2 diabetes presents to their outpatient diabetes education class with their blood glucose log and food journal. They report frustration with their postprandial blood glucose levels after breakfast despite stating that they have been meeting their carbohydrate goal of 30 to 45 g per meal and exercising 30 minutes 5 days per week. The patient's food journal for most breakfasts states: "two scrambled eggs, two slices of toast, one cup coffee, one small apple." What would be the best clarifying question to help determine the discrepancy between the patient's report and the blood glucose log?

    A. "Did you eat whole eggs or egg whites?"
    B. "Was the bread white or wheat?"
    C. "Was the coffee black?"
    D. "What type of apple did you eat?"

135. Current medical nutrition therapy and documentation should be in what format?

    A. Assessment, diagnosis, intervention, monitoring, and evaluation (ADIME)
    B. Subjective, objective, assessment, and plan (SOAP)
    C. Anthropometry, biochemistry, clinical, and diet (ABCD)
    D. Problem, etiology, and signs/symptoms (PES)

136. A patient newly diagnosed with type 2 diabetes presents for a 2-week follow-up. At their last visit, they made a goal to track their dietary intake with a goal of 45 to 60 g of carbohydrates per meal and 0 to 15 g per snack. Their food record shows that a typical day consisted of: breakfast: one cup multigrain Cheerios, one cup skim milk, one banana, 8 oz orange juice, and black coffee; lunch: ham sandwich, small bag of potato chips, and diet soda; dinner: 4 oz grilled steak, one cup broccoli, one cup wild rice, small roll, and unsweetened tea; snack: one whole graham cracker and 1 tbs peanut butter or a small fruit. What would be the best recommendation after reviewing the patient's food record?

A. Eat half the banana at breakfast and save the other half for a snack

B. Reduce intake of "empty calories," including potato chips

C. Consume only one snack per day

D. Substitute leaner options for meat choices

137. A patient presents to their outpatient diabetes prevention class and asks what they can do to help prevent diabetes. They have an A1C of 6.2%, weight of 215 lb, and body mass index (BMI) of 31, and they have not started any diabetes-related medication. What would be an appropriate recommendation?

A. Aim for weight loss of 15 to 20 lb

B. Eliminate carbohydrate intake and increase protein intake

C. Participate in moderate to intense physical activity 45 to 60 minutes per day

D. Initiate insulin when A1C reaches 6.5%

138. A patient brings their 1-week food journal for review. Which of the following recorded lunches meet the patient's carbohydrate goal of 45 to 60 g per meal?

A. "Open face" cold-cut sandwich, one cup chocolate pudding, 1.5 cups grapes, 8 oz sweet tea

B. Two slices from a medium pepperoni pizza, diet soda

C. Chicken caesar salad from a fast-food restaurant, diet soda

D. Hamburger and medium fries from a fast-food restaurant, diet soda

139. Two factors that can interfere with glucose meter accuracy are:

A. Hypoxemia and high-dose vitamin D

B. Hypoxemia and high-dose vitamin C

C. Hyperthyroidism and high-dose vitamin D

D. Hyperthyroidism and high-dose vitamin C

140. When should blood glucose levels be checked with pattern management?

A. Every 4 to 6 hours

B. Fasting before bedtime

C. 1 hour postprandially

D. Fasting and 2 hours postprandially

141. Benefits of a "smart pen" would include:

A. Downloadable data reports

B. Continuous glucose monitoring

C. Increased carbohydrate requirement

D. Replacement of basal insulin

142. An older adult patient with type 2 diabetes presents to an outpatient clinic appointment after 2 years of canceling or no-showing. They have a history of homelessness and state that they are currently living in a shelter after having lived in their car for 6 months. The patient states that they decided to "start watching carbs and taking shots again" but that their plan is not working like it did in the past. The diabetes educator verifies the patient's plan and their understanding of it. The patient empties the contents of their bag on the desk, revealing many boxes of unused insulin and test strips. What factor would most likely contribute to the patient's continued elevated blood glucose levels?

A. Food insecurity and inconsistent carbohydrate intake

B. Inadequate bolus insulin dosing before meals

C. Ineffective insulin and testing strips

D. Inadequate physical activity and weight gain

143. A 17-year-old patient with type 1 diabetes presents with their caregiver to an outpatient follow-up appointment. This discussion becomes tense as the caregiver questions the patient's compliance with taking insulin due to their recent erratic and elevated blood glucose levels. The patient becomes defensive, stating that they "always count carbs and take insulin with meals," and expresses a desire to manage their diabetes plan more independently. What follow-up question might provide insight into the patient's variable blood sugar levels?

A. "Are you sure you haven't missed any doses?"

B. "Are you eating enough carbohydrates with meals?"

C. "How much physical activity are you engaging in each day?"

D. "Are you taking your bolus insulin before or after your meal?"

144. The downloaded report from a patient's continuous glucose monitor (CGM) reveals that the patient's blood glucose levels were within range 90% of the time over the last 2 months. However, the report notes a pattern of middle-of-the-night hypoglycemic episodes. What factor would most likely contribute to these hypoglycemic episodes?

   A. Inadequate carbohydrate intake with dinner
   B. Lack of 15-g carbohydrate snack before bed
   C. Evening alcohol intake
   D. 30-minute afternoon walk

145. While reviewing the blood glucose log of a patient with type 2 diabetes, the diabetes educator notices a pattern of elevated fasting glucose levels. What would be an appropriate recommendation for the patient to help determine the cause of this pattern?

   A. Take an additional blood glucose reading at 3:00 a.m.
   B. Reduce dinner carbohydrate intake by 15 to 30 g
   C. Eliminate alcohol intake in the evening
   D. Initiate 30 to 60 minutes of moderate exercise in the morning

146. An older adult patient with type 2 diabetes reports not checking their blood sugar regularly because it bothers their neuropathy. They also forgot their meter and log book for the second appointment in a row. The patient lives with their adult child, who assists them with following their diabetes care plan. What would be a helpful tool for this patient that would also better allow the diabetes educator and the family member to support the patient more effectively?

   A. Insulin "smart pen"
   B. Automatic blood glucose monitor
   C. 26- to 30-gauge lanceting device
   D. Continuous glucose monitor (CGM)

147. A patient newly diagnosed with type 2 diabetes has completed their diabetes self-management education (DSME) class and reports that they are struggling to "make sense of" their glucometer readings, stay motivated, and find low-cost foods they can eat. What might be an appropriate intervention for this patient?

   A. Ask the patient to repeat the DSME class at another facility
   B. Recommend an online diabetes education class the patient can do from home
   C. Refer the patient to a shared medical appointment
   D. Reassure the patient that better blood glucose control will take time

148. An older adult patient with type 2 diabetes reports difficulty feeling motivated to count carbohydrates and track their blood glucose. They report feeling lonely because they live alone and have no family local to them. What type of support would be most helpful and appropriate for this patient?

    A. Service dog trained in diabetes support
    B. Diabetes support group
    C. Phone application to track diet and exercise
    D. Meal delivery service

149. During an outpatient nutrition therapy appointment, the registered dietitian nutritionist (RDN) calculates and recommends the goal of 30 to 45 g of carbohydrates per meal based on interviewing the patient and accounting for height, weight, and activity level. The RDN proceeds to show the patient sample meal plans that would meet the goal of 30 to 45 g of carbohydrates. After looking at several sample meal plans, the patient states that there is "no way" they could eat such a small amount of carbohydrates and states that they do not want to try. What would be an appropriate initial next step for the RDN?

    A. Maintain recommendation of 30 to 45 g of carbohydrates and note the patient's response in their chart
    B. Explain to the patient that if they eat more carbohydrates their insulin dosage will need to be increased
    C. Request that the patient attempt the proposed goal of 30 to 45 g of carbohydrates per meal for 2 weeks
    D. Work with the patient to determine a carbohydrate goal that the patient feels would be realistic for them

150. A 14-year-old patient recently diagnosed with diabetes attends their final outpatient diabetes education class with their parent. The patient does well in school and has shown a good understanding of their diabetes and management plan. They are very active in extracurricular activities and sports, which leads to a very inconsistent eating and sleeping schedule. The patient's parent expresses confidence that the patient will be able to manage their diabetes successfully. What topic would be beneficial to discuss with the patient's parent?

    A. Focusing on increasing the patient's independent problem-solving skills
    B. Prioritizing diabetes care and reducing the patient's extracurricular activities
    C. Managing the patient's medications until they are an adult
    D. Setting a goal of diabetes management interdependence

151. A local dentist calls the clinic as they have recently had several patients with diabetes who needed to be scheduled for treatment of periodontal disease. The dentist inquires about ways they can partner with the clinic to improve their patients' recoveries. What will the diabetes educator recommend?

A. Refer patients for an outpatient diabetes educator consultation prior to and after treatment

B. Mail educational materials on carbohydrate counting, insulin management, and wound care

C. Create a video for patients to watch at home explaining how positive glucose control promotes healing

D. Refer patients to attend a diabetes self-management education (DSME) course at the local hospital

152. During an outpatient follow-up appointment, a diabetes educator meets with a 16-year-old patient and their parents. The patient was diagnosed 3 years ago with type 1 diabetes but recently has had variable blood glucose readings and several hypoglycemic episodes. The parents state that the patient is not counting carbohydrates or taking insulin at the right times unless reminded. The patient becomes defensive and states that their parents blame them for their high blood sugar levels and do not believe them even when they take their insulin. What concept of parental support likely applies?

A. Interdependence

B. Miscarried helping

C. Active parental involvement

D. Parental reinforcement

153. An adult patient has cystic fibrosis (CF) and diabetes. Referral and communication with which member of the healthcare team is imperative for positive medical outcomes for this patient?

A. Exercise physiologist

B. Oncologist

C. Registered dietitian nutritionist

D. Clinical psychologist

154. During a diabetes prevention class, the diabetes educator shares information about the U.S. Diabetes Prevention Program (USDPP) trial and asks patients to create their own weight loss and physical activity goals. One adult patient in attendance weighs 250 pounds and is 69 inches tall. What would be a realistic weight loss goal, in pounds, for this patient?

A. 5 to 10
B. 13 to 18
C. 20 to 25
D. 23 to 30

155. What was the largest trial that showed lifestyle having a greater impact on diabetes prevention than medication?

A. Da Qing China
B. Finnish Diabetes Prevention Study
C. Japanese Prevention Trials
D. U.S. Diabetes Prevention Program (USDPP)

156. An older adult patient presents for their initial diabetes outpatient consultation. They were recently diagnosed with type 2 diabetes and have a history of hypertension, pulmonary embolism, hypothyroidism, and obesity. In response to the diabetes educator inquiring about their medications, the patient pulls out 10 bottles of prescription pills and supplements and states that they "get mixed up on which ones to take sometimes." What is the patient at risk for?

A. Drug–drug interactions
B. Drug-induced allergic reactions
C. Drug-induced hyperglycemia
D. Medication noncompliance

157. A parent calls the diabetes educator to inform them of a hypoglycemic episode that just occurred while their 10-year-old was at a summer day camp.
While playing outside, the child reported feeling dizzy, and the camp counselor assisted them in checking their blood sugar, which resulted in a reading
of 65 mg/dL. The camp counselor provided the child with a glucose tablet
and a glass of water. After 15 minutes, they rechecked the blood glucose level
and found that it was still 65 mg/dL. The camp staff proceeded to call the
parent to inform them of the situation and ask what their next steps should
be. What would be an appropriate first response?

A. "What type of activity was the child engaged in at the time of their
hypoglycemic episode?"

B. "Call 911 and report that the child is experiencing hypoglycemia and is
not responding to treatment measures."

C. "Tell the counselor to immediately give the child four glucose tablets
and recheck blood sugar in 15 minutes."

D. "The counselor and child should have waited 30 minutes before recheck-
ing to give the tablets more time to increase blood glucose."

158. During a staff meeting, it is brought to the nurse case manager's attention
that many of the staff are struggling to assist their patients with diabetes
who use insulin pumps. What would be the best potential solution?

A. Send out a mandatory webinar on insulin pump directions

B. Assign patients with insulin pumps only to nurses who are experienced
with insulin pumps

C. Instruct nurses to consult the diabetes educator for patients' insulin
pumps

D. Designate a diabetes resource nurse to provide an in-service and mentor
peers on their units

159. The American Diabetes Association (ADA) recommends what medication as
secondary prevention for patients with diabetes and atherosclerotic cardiovascular disease?

A. Aspirin

B. Insulin

C. Metformin

D. Simvastatin

160. If a patient is on a premixed insulin plan or a fixed insulin plan, which of the following statements by the patient would indicate the need for further education?

    A. "I will eat at the same times each day."
    B. "I will eat consistent carbohydrates."
    C. "I will eat when my schedule allows."
    D. "I will be sure that my carbohydrates match the insulin dose."

161. A patient with type 1 diabetes has frequent postprandial spikes, but 3 hours postprandial, the glucose levels normalize. Which of the following would be the cause of these spikes?

    A. Taking insulin 15 minutes before meals
    B. Taking the prescribed insulin-to-carbohydrate ratio
    C. Taking the prescribed insulin postprandial
    D. Taking the insulin 20 minutes before meals

162. An adult patient comes to the clinic with a record of glucose readings that range between 80 and 200 mg/dL. Their A1C is 8.2%. The diabetes educator recommends a blinded continuous glucose monitoring trial. What predominant pattern might be found once the trial is complete?

    A. The patient is having postprandial spikes between 250 and 300 mg/dL
    B. The patient's nocturnal glucose is consistently elevated
    C. The patient is having hyperglycemia in the morning
    D. The patient is having elevated fasting glucose levels

163. An older adult patient with type 2 diabetes takes 15 units of U-500 insulin QID (=300 units) and is eating sweets. When assessed, the patient is found to have nocturnal hypoglycemia and has had a 60 lb (27 kg) weight gain over 5 years, since starting insulin. The A1C is 10%. What immediate interventions could improve the patient's condition?

    A. Educate the patient on a diet low in simple carbohydrates and reduce insulin by 50%
    B. Recommend reduction in the insulin by 25% and add sitagliptin 100 mg
    C. Recommend that the patient start a glucagon-like peptide 1 receptor (GLP-1) agonist and reduce insulin by 30%
    D. Educate the patient on a low-calorie diet and reduce insulin by 25%

164. An adult patient with suspected type 1 diabetes has been having urticaria at the insulin injection site, presenting with a pruritic rash and erythema surrounding the site. An insulin allergy is suspected. The educator refers the patient to a dermatologist. What diagnostic tool will be used to confirm this condition?

   A. Blood test
   B. Intradermal skin testing
   C. Skin prick test
   D. Patch test

165. A 17-year-old patient has been mostly independent in managing their diabetes. The last A1C was 12%, and insulin has been given mostly post meal due to fear of having hypoglycemia while around friends. An unknown number of glucose checks are being done daily as the patient has multiple glucometers. In collaboration with the patient and their parents, what assessment question would be the most appropriate?

   A. Is the patient interested in a continuous glucose meter (CGM)?
   B. How many times a day is the patient checking their glucose?
   C. Why isn't the patient testing their glucose levels regularly?
   D. Can the parents get more involved with glucose testing?

166. A patient underwent 3 days of blinded continuous glucose monitoring (CGM) and kept close records of insulin dosing, food intake, and glucose levels throughout the day. The downloaded CGM tracings showed large increases in glucose 3 hours after eating dinner for 4 days. This information was not reflected in the patient's records. The amount of morning hyperglycemia was related to the postprandial dinner glucose levels. How could the patient demonstrate these effects using glucose finger sticks in the future, without the use of a CGM?

   A. Instruct the patient to test 1 hour postprandial
   B. Have the patient check glucose levels before dinner and 2 hours postprandial
   C. Have the patient check glucose levels 3 hours postprandial
   D. Have the patient check glucose levels 2 hours postprandial

167. A 6-year-old patient is diagnosed with type 1 diabetes. When educating the family and the patient, what is the best glucose monitoring schedule to recommend when taking insulin three or more times daily?

A. Before each meal and as needed
B. Fasting, before meals, bedtime, and 2 a.m.
C. Before meals and at bedtime
D. Before meals, bedtime, and fasting

168. An older adult patient who lives alone is being discharged from the hospital on insulin. The patient is cognitively unable to learn insulin-to-carbohydrate ratio, so a fixed mealtime insulin is ordered along with a basal insulin. Which of the following instructional methods can the educator use that would benefit the patient most?

A. Review survival skills verbally and have the patient repeat back the dosing instructions
B. Write down the doses, verbally tell the patient the doses, and call the patient in the morning
C. Contact a friend or family member to help the patient
D. Review the information with the patient verbally on their discharge summary

169. An adult patient with type 2 diabetes and low cardiovascular risk factors has a low-density lipoprotein (LDL) of 156 mg/dL, triglycerides of 125 mg/dL, high-density lipoprotein (HDL) of 60 mg/dL, blood pressure (BP) of 125/75 mmHg, and A1C of 6.4 % and is of optimal weight. The patient exercises regularly. After assessing the patient, what can the educator do to set optimal goals for this patient?

A. Instruct the patient to reduce their fat intake to 50 g per day
B. Instruct the patient to increase their exercise to 150 minutes per week
C. Notify the provider and request that the patient be prescribed a statin
D. Advise the patient to continue with current lifestyle choices

170. The patient has a prescription for premixed 70/30 neutral protamine hagedorn (NPH)/regular insulin. What goals can be set for the patient to promote euglycemia?

A. The patient can take their insulin every 12 hours
B. The patient can take their insulin 30 minutes before meals
C. The patient can take insulin 30 minutes before breakfast and dinner
D. The patient can take insulin as directed on the prescription

171. An 80-year-old patient with congestive heart failure, controlled hypertension, and atrial fibrillation is newly diagnosed with type 2 diabetes with an initial A1C of 9.5%. Following the educator's assessment, what lifestyle goals would be realistic for the patient to meet?

    A. A1C to be less than 7% within 3 months

    B. Postprandial glucose readings to be less than 180 mg/dL

    C. To begin an exercise program at the senior center

    D. A1C to be less than 8% within 3 months

172. A patient who has had type 1 diabetes for many years tells their diabetes educator that they know basic self-monitoring of blood glucose (SMBG) skills, including when to check blood sugars, recommended ranges, how to interpret results, and when to contact a healthcare provider. What would be an appropriate next topic for the diabetes educator to discuss with the patient?

    A. Finger site selection

    B. Hypoglycemia and hyperglycemia definitions

    C. How the chemicals in the strip react with glucose

    D. Pattern management

173. A patient with type 1 diabetes who is experiencing homelessness is admitted to the hospital in diabetic ketoacidosis (DKA). Upon assessment, it is revealed that the patient has access to insulin. However, there is no proper storage for the insulin, and it may have been damaged by being exposed to heat. What is the most imperative educational goal to be set for this patient regarding insulin storage?

    A. Allowing insulin to be at room temperature while open is okay

    B. Insulin should be stored in the dark at all times

    C. Avoid exposing insulin to temperatures above 86°F

    D. Keep insulin between 36°F and 46°F at all times

174. Which of the following is the most effective strategy for assessing the learning needs of a patient?

    A. Inquire about the patient's level of understanding and what they want to learn

    B. Ask the patient how long they have had diabetes

    C. Have the patient complete a Patient Health Questionnaire-9 (PHQ-9)

    D. Include family members and caregivers in the discussion

175. What reading level is appropriate for written diabetes educational materials for most patients?

A. Twelfth grade or higher

B. Fifth to sixth grade

C. Second to third grade

D. Customized to each patient's reading level

176. A patient with type 1 diabetes meets with their healthcare provider, and they establish that the patient should monitor their blood sugar more often. What information should be gathered from the patient before setting a goal for self-monitoring of blood glucose (SMBG)?

A. The patient's meal and activity schedule

B. How often the patient currently performs SMBG

C. The patient's most recent A1C

D. The patient's support network

177. Parents of a 10-year-old patient with newly diagnosed type 1 diabetes are learning how to calculate rapid-acting insulin doses for their child based on carbohydrate ratio and sensitivity factor. What is the most effective way for their diabetes educator to help them learn?

A. Explain the 1800 rule to the parents

B. Explain to the parents how to test the child's carbohydrate ratio

C. Provide written materials to the parents that explain the concepts of carbohydrate ratio and insulin sensitivity factor

D. Provide scenarios of meals and premeal blood glucose values and ask the parents to calculate proper insulin doses

178. When is a patient more likely to see significant differences in continuous glucose monitoring (CGM) measures of interstitial glucose and plasma glucose?

A. When the sensor is close to expiration

B. When the sensor is worn on the back of the arm

C. When glucose levels are rising or falling rapidly

D. When glucose levels are falling rapidly

179. What type of insulin is delivered through insulin pump therapy?

A. Long-acting and rapid-acting insulin

B. Long-acting insulin

C. Intermediate-acting insulin

D. Rapid-acting insulin

180. A patient with type 1 diabetes comes in for a follow-up visit. The patient uses an insulin pump, and their pump download shows that they often have short periods of hyperglycemia followed by hypoglycemia with meals. What change is recommended for this patient?

A. The carbohydrate ratio needs to be strengthened

B. The patient should be instructed to pre-bolus before meals

C. The basal rate must be increased before the meal and then decreased after the meal

D. The sensitivity needs to be strengthened

181. A patient with uncontrolled diabetes for many years shares that they want to improve their health but feel incapable of making the necessary changes to do so. What barrier to learning is this patient exhibiting?

A. Low motivation

B. Numeracy

C. Low self-efficacy

D. Noncompliance

182. What term is used to describe a sense of being overwhelmed or a feeling of failure or frustration in an individual with diabetes?

A. Denial

B. Anxiety

C. Diabetes distress

D. Depression

183. A patient with type 1 diabetes states that they take 5 to 10 units of lispro (Humalog) per meal depending on how much they eat but do not account for their blood sugar. Their progress note from their physician states that they have a sensitivity factor of 1:50 > 150. Which issue may warrant further assessment when working with this patient?

A. Numeracy

B. Diabetes distress

C. Memory problems

D. Reading literacy

184. A patient states that they have been making their lunch at least 3 days each week instead of going to fast-food restaurants and have been going to the gym at least 4 days a week for the past 2 months. Which stage of change is this patient demonstrating?

    A. Maintenance
    B. Preparation
    C. Contemplation
    D. Action

185. The transtheoretical model of change suggests that people go through five specific stages when changing behaviors. Which stages does the model include?

    A. Preparation, action, revision, maintenance, and termination
    B. Precontemplation, contemplation, preparation, action, and maintenance
    C. Contemplation, skills acquisition, preparation, action, and maintenance
    D. Precontemplation, preparation, action, self-evaluation, and maintenance

186. A patient with newly diagnosed diabetes states that they do not want to take their medications or perform glucose checks because they do not want to acknowledge their diagnosis. What intervention is most appropriate for this patient?

    A. Assess cognitive capacity
    B. Refer to endocrinology
    C. Provide continuous glucose monitoring training
    D. Provide one-on-one education

187. A patient shares that they intentionally skip their insulin if their blood sugar is less than 150 because they say this is a low level for them. What is most important to address with this patient?

    A. Discuss relative hypoglycemia
    B. Review the rule of 15
    C. Instruct them to have a bedtime snack
    D. Educate them on hypoglycemic unawareness

4. PRACTICE EXAM   161

188. What counterregulatory hormone causes rebound hyperglycemia following untreated or undertreated hypoglycemia?

  A. Amylin
  B. Glucagon
  C. Incretin
  D. Insulin

189. A 16-year-old patient with diabetes that was previously well controlled has recently developed worsening blood glucose control. Their parents are worried and have asked the patient to report all of their blood sugars to them, which the patient has resisted. What is the most appropriate intervention?

  A. Ask the patient what they need from family members regarding their diabetes management
  B. Encourage the patient to self-manage their diabetes independently
  C. Prescribe a continuous glucose monitoring device that allows data sharing
  D. Educate the patient and the family about the complications that can result from worsening control

190. A patient with type 1 diabetes is about to celebrate their birthday and asks their provider how drinking alcohol will affect their diabetes. What is the best response?

  A. Advise the patient to abstain from alcohol regardless of the occasion
  B. Tell the patient to take rapid-acting insulin before drinking to cover the carbohydrates in alcohol
  C. Educate the patient on the direct and indirect effects of alcohol on blood glucose levels
  D. Ensure that the patient has a prescription for glucagon

191. Which class of oral medications for diabetes has a higher risk of hypoglycemia when paired with alcohol?

  A. Sulfonylureas
  B. Thiazolidinediones
  C. Biguanides
  D. Sodium-glucose co-transporter 2 (SGLT2) inhibitors

192. A 14-year-old patient and their parents meet with a diabetes educator to develop a plan to help ensure that the patient can independently self-manage their diabetes prior to leaving for college in 4 years. Where is a good place to start?

    A. Review the patient's current self-care skills
    B. Encourage the patient to begin independently managing their diabetes as soon as possible
    C. Transfer the patient to an adult provider
    D. Have the patient attend healthcare appointments independently

193. A patient with uncontrolled type 1 diabetes shares that they feel burdened by having to manage their disease and continue to miss multiple insulin doses despite meeting with a diabetes educator for one-on-one education. What is the appropriate next intervention for this patient?

    A. Enroll them in group education sessions
    B. Refer them to a behavioral health provider
    C. Review the complications of uncontrolled diabetes
    D. Prescribe mixed insulin twice a day to reduce their number of injections

194. A patient who has had diabetes for more than 10 years reports multiple episodes of severe hypoglycemia during the course of the disease. What is most important for the provider to assess in this patient?

    A. Injuries from falls
    B. Depression
    C. Adherence to medications
    D. Cognitive capacity

195. A patient who was diagnosed with type 2 diabetes more than 10 years ago is unable to control their blood sugar despite taking three oral medications. The physician prescribes insulin, and their blood sugars normalize within 2 days. Which is the best explanation for the change in their condition?

    A. Progressive insulin resistance
    B. Decline in beta-cell function
    C. Autoimmunity
    D. Decreased incretin effect

196. A young adult patient with diabetes goes to the gym and engages in 60 minutes of moderate aerobic exercise followed by resistance workouts every Friday, Saturday, and Sunday. During the rest of the week, they do not engage in exercise. What can be assessed about the patient's activity needs?

A. They should add another 30 to 60 minutes of activity to their week

B. They should not exercise more than 2 days in a row to prevent injuries

C. They should add 1 more day of resistance training during the week

D. They should not go 2 or more consecutive days without activity

197. A patient with type 2 diabetes takes fixed insulin doses at breakfast, lunch, and dinner. They state that they may have eggs and a slice of toast for breakfast 1 day and pancakes, hash browns, and fruit the next day. For lunch, they may have a sandwich or a salad. For dinner, they may have pasta with garlic bread or salmon and vegetables. What dietary education is most important for this patient?

A. Education regarding the benefits of a low-carbohydrate diet

B. Information about consistent patterns of carbohydrate intake

C. Information about a Mediterranean-style eating plan

D. Education on the glycemic impact of carbohydrates, fats, and proteins

198. A patient with diabetes and proliferative diabetic retinopathy states that they want to start weight training. Which recommendation would be appropriate for this patient?

A. They should try to engage in two to three sessions of resistance training per week on nonconsecutive days

B. They should also include flexibility training and balance training two to three times per week

C. They should schedule a consultation with an ophthalmologist

D. They should be referred to a cardiologist

199. The diabetes educator and the patient are reviewing medications that can cause glucose levels to rise. The patient demonstrates understanding when they identify which medication as a non–glucose rising medication?

A. Glucocorticoids

B. Thiazide diuretics

C. Risperidone

D. Quinolones

200. Which features identify key differences in patients with diabetic ketoacidosis (DKA) versus patients with hyperosmolar hyperglycemic syndrome (HHS)?

    A. Age, duration of symptoms, and glucose levels

    B. Age, sodium concentration, and potassium concentration

    C. Ketone bodies, bicarbonate concentration, and age

    D. Bicarbonate concentration, age, and sodium concentration

Practice Exam Answers With Rationales

1. C) Decrease the lipid values of the patients

Accreditation standards must include quality measures that measure the effectiveness of behavioral and participant outcome goals; decreasing the lipid values of the patients is an example of an outcome goal. Increasing attendance, decreasing documentation errors, and increasing patient satisfaction are goals unrelated to patient health outcomes.

2. A) To identify blood glucose goals

Being able to identify blood glucose levels is a good objective because it communicates the instructor's intent well and leaves little room for interpretation. Learning objectives often begin with "define," "discuss," "describe," "list," or "state." Terms such as "believe," "acknowledge," and "understand" start objectives that are not as clearly measurable or observable.

3. D) Role-playing activity

Role-playing is an appropriate format for a patient needing to practice and gain confidence in situations such as eating out and social events. Reading booklets, web-based learning, and discussion will provide tips and enhance problem-solving skills but will not be as immediately applicable in the day-to-day situations with which this patient is struggling.

4. D) A qualified representative of the school district

A qualified representative of the school district is a professional who has the skills and knowledge to assess needs and provide services for the child and should be included in the discussion. The school district representative can be a support in accessing and providing needed tools and resources for the child. An attorney, physical education teacher, and qualified occupational therapist are not necessary participants.

5. B) Problem-solving

AADE7 behavior change topics include problem-solving along with being active, eating, taking medications, appropriate monitoring, reducing risks, and living with diabetes. Knowledge skills would occur before the class while assessing learning. Smoking cessation and weight loss are specific clinical improvement measures that are outcomes of behavior change.

6. D) Liraglutide

Liraglutide is the only approved glucagon-like peptide-1 (GLP-1) used as a specific weight management medication. Fluoxetine and triamterene are high-risk medication additives often found in dietary weight loss supplements and have warnings from the U.S. Food and Drug Administration (FDA) as contaminants. Exenatide, also a GLP-1, can help with weight loss but is not approved as a weight-loss drug.

7. D) Establish the patient's current skills of self-management

When transitions in care occur, the diabetes educator needs to provide support for the patient to maintain independence as part of assisting in establishing a transition plan. Therefore, it is important to understand the patient's skills of self-management. Reinforcing the importance of nutrition and discussing risk reduction and prevention of complications may not be necessary if the patient's self-management is determined to be optimal since this could indicate they already understand nutrition and risk reduction. The transition in care does not necessarily lead to depression or diabetes distress.

8. A) Importance of routine checkups

Any type of healthcare provider, including a nurse assistant, can advise patients on the importance of routine checkups as well as metabolic control, control of cardiovascular risk factors, healthy lifestyle, the benefits of comprehensive team care, and self-exams for foot and dental problems. A certified diabetes educator is uniquely qualified to educate patients on techniques for injecting insulin, blood glucose monitoring schedules, and ketone testing, all of which require specialized knowledge, training, and skill. The nurse assistant is not qualified to provide these types of education.

9. D) Reading literacy

The patient may have problems with reading literacy. Not being able to provide names but providing descriptions of medications is often a sign of low reading literacy. A concern with health literacy would suggest that the patient may know the names of medications but not understand what they are meant to treat. Because the patient can describe the shape and color, there is little evidence of a visual barrier. Numeracy problems would be more evident if there were issues with understanding dosing.

10. C) Dapagliflozin
Dapagliflozin is a sodium-glucose cotransporter 2 inhibitor and has the established disadvantage of causing urinary tract infections. This adverse effect has a causal relationship to the effect of dapagliflozin leading to increased urinary glucose excretion. Atorvastatin, metformin, and lisinopril have other adverse effects but are not associated with urinary tract infections.

11. D) Ability to recognize and report symptoms
The patient should be assessed to determine ability to recognize and report symptoms. In considering age-related skills, a child of 9 years should be able to recognize and report symptoms. However, the child's ability to be aware of symptoms at all times, adjust insulin as needed, and treat episodes may not occur until a few years later, according to studies on age and diabetes self-management skills.

12. C) Monitor before and after all meals
The patient needs to monitor before and after all meals. Premeal and postmeal glucose readings are critical to determine the efficiency of both short- and long-acting insulin. Monitoring only before meals or at varied times or maintaining current monitoring is not appropriate because these would not adequately evaluate glucose control and treatment effectiveness.

13. B) Changes to carbohydrate intake at breakfast
The patient's log indicates that they need to be evaluated for changes to carbohydrate intake at breakfast. The log provides evidence that the greatest concern is postbreakfast hyperglycemia. An evaluation for carbohydrates and possible changes to carbohydrate intake would be helpful. Any other conclusion would require more results and data before evaluating trends and interventions.

14. B) The patient has not met the goals for reducing risks
This patient has not met the goals for reducing risks. An eye exam would fall under risk-reducing self-care behavior. Because the eye exam has not been completed, the goal is not met. A new or adjusted goal would be necessary. The patient has made goals for reducing risks and for monitoring and taking medication, and there is enough information to evaluate their efforts.

15. D) Identifying appropriate food when eating out

At age 11 years, it is appropriate for the patient's learning goals to transition to a higher level of learning about healthy eating and how to make healthy choices. Identifying appropriate food when eating out is an appropriate goal. Altering food intake, creating a meal plan, and adjusting insulin doses will be more appropriate in a few years when the patient is a teenager.

16. A) Proper and consistent nutrition habits

An appropriate topic is education on consistent nutrition habits. Consistent nutrition habits are an American Diabetes Association education recommendation to include as a discharge area of knowledge. Proper nutrition is essential to wound healing and preventing future diabetes-related wounds and infections. Complications of diabetes, psychosocial factors in managing diabetes, and review of home glucose logs are topics discussed in formal diabetes self-management education services, not at hospital discharge, and are less specific to the patient's condition.

17. C) Prescriptions

The concern is how the patient will pay for prescriptions. Medicare Part D is an additional prescription drug benefit. Medicare Parts A and B cover medical services such as home healthcare, supplies, and education.

18. C) 9

The patient should take 9 units to cover both the correction factor and the meal. They are 90 points above their premeal goal of 100. Their correction factor is 1 unit to lower their glucose by 30 points. They need 3 units to correct by 90 points to their target goal. In addition to their correction units, they need 1 unit for every 10 carbs to make 6 units for the 60-g meal. To correct with 3 units and 6 units for the meal is a total of 9 units. The correction factor is only covered by 3 units; 6 units is needed for the carb-to-insulin ratio, and 12 units is too much.

19. A) The patient has latent autoimmune diabetes in adults (LADA) and should begin insulin therapy

The patient has LADA and needs to start insulin therapy. LADA is a form of diabetes with a pathophysiology of late-onset beta cell failure that typically occurs at age 35 or older. Treatment will need to transition to insulin despite some evidence that people with LADA may remain insulin independent for years. Therefore, increasing oral therapy is not likely to be beneficial. MODY develops before age 35, so MODY is not the likely cause for this patient's condition.

20. A) Review two short videos on exercise options for seniors
Providing options and helping the patient formulate a list of possible activities will help the patient move toward behavioral goals. By reviewing two short videos on exercise for seniors, the patient will see that others like them are capable of exercising successfully. A handout on senior gyms does not address their concerns about performing the exercises. Shoes and foot care may be a conversation for a later visit but do not relate to the patient's immediate concerns. Demonstrating chair exercises shows limited options and is not collaborative in helping the patient fully explore exercise options.

21. A) They may be pricking the middle of their fingertip
The patient is likely pricking the middle of their fingertip where all of the nerve endings are. They should try putting their palms flat and fingers pressed together and testing along the edges that are now visible. A smaller-gauge lancet would likely help reduce pain. Not milking their fingers and being dehydrated would be reasons for inadequate sample size, not pain.

22. C) Six
The patient's meal included six carbohydrate choices. A 1/3-cup serving of pasta is one carbohydrate choice, so 1 cup of pasta is the equivalent of three carbohydrate choices, the piece of garlic bread is one carbohydrate, and the yogurt and fruit are two carbohydrates for a total of six carbohydrate choices.

23. B) Suggest recumbent cycling as a potential safe exercise
Recumbent cycling is a potential safe exercise for this patient. Education should focus on hypotension, not hypertension, during physical exercise. Rapid-acting insulin may need to be delayed until after exercise. Warm environments are a risk and should not be recommended.

24. B) The teaching was ineffective for the patient's learning needs, and they need a new learning plan
The teaching was ineffective for the patient's learning needs, and they need a new learning plan. Part of evaluation is to evaluate effectiveness of teaching. This patient's being overwhelmed and unable to demonstrate learning suggests they have not achieved learning objectives and need ongoing planning for learning goals. This situation does not reflect any concerns with the class's instructional style. There has been no meaningful progress toward behavioral or learning goals.

25. C) Adhering to taking medications

Adherence to taking medications is an appropriate intermediate outcome to measure in this patient. Intermediate outcomes are good measures of behavior change, such as medication adherence. Understanding medication side effects is a desired immediate outcome measurement that involves learning, knowledge, and skills. Measuring the reduction in A1C and tracking improvement in quality of life are postintermediate and long-term outcomes because they show clinical indicators and health status changes that take time to measure.

26. A) Ask the patient to calculate carbohydrates from a beverage label

The best way to evaluate this patient's learning is to have them calculate carbohydrates from a beverage label. Having the patient teach back negative effects of sugared beverages would not demonstrate learning of alternative drink choices. Assessing drink choices and reviewing glucose logs are more consistent with evaluating behavioral changes and behavior goals that would come after meeting the learning goals.

27. A) "Monitor your glucose frequently to check for hypoglycemia."

Autonomic neuropathy results when diabetes has begun to affect the autonomic nervous systems. Symptoms include cardiac irregularities (tachycardia, bradycardia, hypotension), edema, paradoxical supine hypertension, heat intolerance, and gastrointestinal and genitourinary dysfunction. Hypoglycemia, therefore, becomes a higher risk due to lack of awareness and lack of symptom response, so it is important for the patient to measure their glucose level often. Wearing shoes to protect the feet would be advice more appropriate for a patient who presents with sensorimotor neuropathy, which involves sensory nerves and often presents with pain, aching, burning, and stabbing sensations in the limbs. Mononeuropathy occurs most frequently in older patients. Pain is a primary symptom and results from vascular obstruction; it is often sudden in onset and resolves spontaneously, unlike autonomic neuropathy. Large-fiber neuropathy is a type of sensorimotor neuropathy that presents with lower extremity cramping pain and altered sensation when walking, which results in ataxia and risk of falls. Although orthostatic hypotension can cause a patient to fall upon standing, changing the home layout will not prevent this, so this instruction is more appropriate for a patient with large-fiber neuropathy.

28. B) Look for three or more consistent patterns

The patient should do nothing related to the current pattern but should look for three or more consistent patterns. High blood glucose readings at the same time of day for 3 or more days in 1 week or low readings on 2 or more days can indicate a pattern. The two nonconsecutive patterns do not necessarily support needing to adjust exercise or meals or increase the patient's insulin. Two readings do not provide enough information to make changes.

29. C) Celiac disease

The patient should be tested for celiac disease. Celiac disease is an autoimmune bowel disease identified by an abnormal immune response to gluten in the diet. Celiac disease has a higher prevalence among those with type 1 diabetes and should therefore be a consideration for screening in patients with type 1 diabetes. Addison's disease and Graves' disease are also considered autoimmune diseases that are frequent comorbidities of type 1 diabetes, but they are thyroid-related diseases without gastrointestinal symptoms. Crohn's disease is an inflammatory disease of the digestive system; however, there are no current recommendations for concurrent screening with type 1 diabetes.

30. A) "What makes this change important to you?"

"What makes this change important to you?" is an appropriate response when using motivational interviewing, which uses active listening and facilitating questions to identify feelings and discrepancies in acting on those feelings. Asking about risks would demonstrate using the health belief model, a model that helps the educator understand behaviors from a point of susceptibility, severity, benefits, barriers, and self-efficacy. Asking about environment, such as work or home, is consistent with the social cognitive theory, which recognizes factors that can influence behaviors and then lead to methods in behavior change. Asking directly about feelings fits more closely with the empowerment-based behavior change protocol that engages reflecting, discussing, solving problems, responding, and choosing. While discussing what makes the change important to the patient also considers the patient's feelings, it is better to focus on the patient's motivations to make proactive choices rather than simply their reaction to a failure to meet goals.

31. B) "Large amounts of meat or fat can make your blood glucose higher, and you may need more insulin."

Large amounts of meat or fat can increase blood glucose, and more insulin may be required. In one study, participants needed an average of 42% more insulin following a high-fat meal compared with a low-fat meal. Despite additional insulin, blood glucose remained higher for 5 to 10 hours after consumption of a high-fat meal. Large amounts of meat may not be good for the patient's heart, but it will also impact blood glucose. The protein will not make blood glucose lower. The educator should not encourage the diabetes patient to eat a low-carb diet with large amounts of meat.

32. C) "I would prefer that you test your glucose fasting and after meals on 2 days of the week."

Testing glucose while fasting and after meals on 2 days of the week would use about the same number of strips per month but would provide a more consistent understanding of how the patient's glycemic control has been. Telling the patient that they should test their glucose three times a day, even though they have already indicated that they cannot afford to do so, is unrealistic. Asking them whether they can cut back in other areas of their budget is condescending and unsupportive.

33. B) "How much help do you need with cooking?"

Asking how much help the patient needs with cooking assesses their ability to perform activities of daily living. The abilities to cook, do laundry, and dress oneself are examples of activities of daily living. Asking about the ability to read a newspaper, hear the TV, or walk without becoming short of breath, or about the number of recent falls, is assessing other physical capabilities and limitations.

34. B) She may need to be assessed for disordered eating behaviors

An appropriate consideration would be to consider a further referral to assess for disordered eating behaviors. Women who have type 1 diabetes are more than twice as likely to develop an eating disorder than women of the same age who do not have diabetes. Diabetes distress occurs as a result of struggling with the continued demands of diabetes, which is not the case with this patient. Adjustment disorder tends to present at the time of diagnosis. A discussion of continuous glucose monitoring would be more appropriate if the patient demonstrated more control over her diabetes.

35. B) "Breakfast may help glucose control by adding consistency to your meal plan."

The patient should be advised that breakfast may help glucose control by adding consistency to their meal plan. The diabetes educator should not encourage the patient to skip meals, have a high-protein breakfast, or exercise on an empty stomach in the morning.

36. B) "It is really calorie restriction that helps improve glycemic control."

Vegetarian diets are one of many diets studied. A consensus recommendation is that vegetarian diets are no better at improving glycemic control unless the diet also considers calorie reduction and supports weight loss. Vegetarian diets are not more successful than other diets. The DASH diet demonstrates a meal pattern that can aid in blood pressure control and cardiovascular health, but there is limited evidence that the DASH diet supports diabetes management. Gluten-free foods should not be encouraged unless the patient has a history of celiac disease. Celiac disease is an immune-mediated disorder that has increased incidence among people with type 1 diabetes; it leads to intestinal damage when gluten is ingested.

37. A) They need to reduce sodium in their diet

The patient has microalbuminuria and needs to reduce sodium intake in their diet. Albuminuria is normal at <30 mg/24 hr. Microalbuminuria is a range between 30 and 299 mg/24 hr, and macroalbuminuria is any result of more than 300 mg/24 hr. Chronic kidney disease is measured by glomerular filtration rate (GFR), not albuminuria. However, there is a clear relationship between elevated albuminuria and a decline in GFR. Salt reduction has been demonstrated to be an effective way to control blood pressure and thus aid in the treatment of developing diabetic kidney disease. Reducing protein is the focus of much research, but studies have not shown that a restricted protein diet at the level of microalbuminuria reduces the risk of further kidney function decline and can lead to malnutrition. Protein, however, is a consideration for careful planning for predialysis advanced diabetic kidney disease. Potassium is also a potential area of further study, but at present there is little specific evidence for restrictions or increases in those nutrients relative to developing kidney disease. The patient's results do not fall in the normal albuminuria range, and so they will need to make changes.

38. A) "Are you using real crabmeat or imitation crab?"
An important emphasis on glycemic control is helping the patient learn how to monitor carbohydrate intake. Imitation crab contains 11 to 16 g of carbohydrate per one-half cup because of added sweeteners and wheat starch. If this patient is having two crab cakes, each containing one-half cup of artificial crabmeat, that is two carbohydrate choices. The slice of bread would make it three carbo-hydrate choices. The melon would make the total four carbohydrate choices. Altogether, the patient is consuming approximately 60 g of carbohydrates at din-ner. Margarine on the vegetables or tartar sauce on the crab cakes would add very little carbohydrate.

39. B) "Large amounts of cinnamon are possibly toxic to the liver."
Cinnamon contains a substance called coumarin, which can cause liver damage in doses over 6 g a day. Just because a supplement is "natural" doesn't necessarily make it safe for use, especially for people taking medication or who have health concerns. Cinnamon is rich in flavonoids and might help to prevent cancer. There is no evidence that cinnamon affects the kidneys.

40. B) "Focusing on the types of fat rather than reducing all fat can be more beneficial."
Current guidelines support focusing on the types of fat rather than the total amount of fat overall to improve one's diet and health. A low-fat diet is not neces-sarily better. Total fat distribution recommendations fall between 20% and 35% of daily caloric intake with a focus on consuming mono- and polyunsaturated fats and reducing saturated fats and avoiding trans fats. Supplements overall are not as beneficial as good food choices.

41. D) Six
The patient ate six carbohydrate choices at breakfast. Carbohydrate choices are in portion sizes of 15 g of carbohydrate. One slice of toast is 15 g. Half of a large banana is 15 g. One-half cup of juice is 15 g. The breakfast total is six.

42. A) A genetic defect affecting beta cell function
Maturity-onset diabetes of the young is a genetic defect affecting beta cell func-tion. Type 1 diabetes is an autoimmune destruction of the beta cells. Insulin resis-tance is associated with type 2 diabetes. Cushing's disease, pheochromocytoma, and acromegaly are associated with hormonal disorder types of diabetes.

43. C) 48

The patient would bolus 48 units. One carbohydrate count is considered 15 g. According to this patient's carbohydrate-to-insulin ratio, the patient is to have 12 units of insulin for every count of carbohydrates. To determine how many insulin units the patient would bolus for a 60-g carbohydrate meal, the patient would multiply 60 g by 12 g/insulin unit to get 720 g, and divide it by 15 g. This results in 48 insulin units for this meal. The 12-unit and 24-unit boluses are not enough for 60 g of carbohydrates, and 72 g is more than necessary.

44. A) "Aim to maintain portion control when you do have meals."

Binge eating can be a risk when fasting patients break their fasts, affecting glucose levels more than the fasting does. Therefore, the patient should be advised to focus on portion control when they do eat. Advising the patient to increase exercise can be a risk factor for dehydration and hypoglycemia. Taking oral medications may be considered breaking the fast, and the patient may wish to opt for temporary medication adjustments. Checking blood glucose levels is important, but not just after a meal. When fasting, the patient should be advised to be aware of signs and symptoms of high and low glucose levels and check more often.

45. D) "How are you correcting your hypoglycemia?"

Many individuals with hypoglycemia do not follow the 15-15 rule (eat 15 grams of carbohydrate, then wait 15 minutes) and instead consume a large amount of carbohydrate in a very short period of time in an effort to feel better, a practice that can cause weight gain. Metformin does not cause weight gain, regardless of the dosage. Depression might be a cause of weight gain, but this should not be the first inquiry since hypoglycemia management should first be assessed. Asking the patient what their weight goal is will not help to determine concrete steps to stop the weight gain, which is what the patient most needs at this time.

46. D) Acarbose

Acarbose will have an immediate effect on blood glucose levels. Januvia and metformin may take 1 to 2 weeks to work. Rosiglitazone will take longer than 2 weeks to have an effect on blood glucose.

47. D) They should have used a finger-stick reading rather than the continuous monitor

The patient should have used a finger-stick reading rather than relying on their continuous glucose monitor. Continuous glucose monitors measure glucose in the fat below the skin and not in the blood. Because of this, they take a long time to show a blood glucose rise after hypoglycemia has been treated. It is better to use a finger-stick reading in this case. Half a cup of apple juice or a third of a cup of grape juice contains the same amount of carbohydrate. The correct amount to treat hypoglycemia is 15 to 20 g of carbohydrate, the amount in both the glucose tablets and the juice. The 15-15 rule states that you treat hypoglycemia with around 15 g of carbohydrate and then test again 15 minutes later, not 30 minutes later.

48. B) Sugar alcohols are lower in calories because they are poorly absorbed and can cause digestive distress

Sugar alcohols are lower in calories because they are poorly absorbed and can cause digestive distress. Sugar alcohols are considered reduced-calorie, not non-nutritive. Even if a food is labeled "no added sugar" or "sugar-free," the calories and carbohydrates in the food must be counted. Although it is true that some sugar alcohols come from fruits and berries, their nutritional value is not equal to a serving of fruit.

49. B) Have a snack plan to avoid low blood sugars

The patient should have a snack plan to avoid low blood sugars. Hypoglycemia can be an added risk when traveling due to many factors, such as uncertain eating schedule, stress, or extra activity. Staying on a rigid schedule with insulin is not recommended because varying meal times and types of foods may require adjustment to normalize glucose levels. Glucose levels should be tested more frequently, not just when necessary. Medications do not have to be sent ahead, but learning Transportation Security Administration (TSA) rules and planning ahead for medication packing is recommended.

50. C) The patient may need medication dose changes for chronic kidney disease

The patient may need medication dose changes for chronic kidney disease as indicated by the glomerular filtration rate of 40. Many oral medications for diabetes require glomerular filtration rate dose adjustments. Glucose levels of 90 to 130 mg/dL are good target ranges, and medications should not be reduced. Desirable cholesterol levels are total cholesterol <200 mg/dL, low-density lipoprotein <70 mg/dL, and triglycerides <150 mg/dL. The patient's levels are within desirable ranges, which would indicate compliance with cholesterol medications.

51. B) E-cigarettes have not been shown to be an effective way to quit

E-cigarettes have not been shown to be an effective way to quit. According to the 2022 American Diabetes Association standards of care, no individual should be advised to use e-cigarettes as a recreational drug or as a way to stop smoking. Further research is needed to fully establish their safety and long-term effects. E-cigarettes are currently not included as part of pharmacologic intervention for smoking cessation and therefore are not considered a good alternative to a nicotine patch.

52. C) Rotating insulin injection sites

Localized lipohypertrophy is the accumulation of fat under the skin. It is often seen in people with diabetes who give injections in the same spot repeatedly, resulting in a buildup of fat and scar tissue. It has been estimated that half of all people with type 1 diabetes experience localized lipohypertrophy, but rotating injection sites can help prevent this. Not reusing needles is best for hygiene and injection comfort, as dull needles can be painful and unclean. Intramuscular injection is a concern with needle size and insertion technique, not lipohypertrophy. Changing needle sizes would be associated with avoiding intramuscular injection, not lipohypertrophy.

53. A) Kidney disease

Kidney disease often manifests as poor appetite, weakness, trouble concentrating, and fluid retention. Itchy skin, dark urine, chronic fatigue, a swollen abdomen, and discolored skin and eyes are symptoms of liver disease. Shortness of breath, edema, swelling in the abdomen and legs, and wheezing are symptoms of congestive heart failure. Slurred speech, loss of memory, paralysis, and numbness or tingling are symptoms of a stroke.

54. B) Before driving and at regular intervals

Patients who use either insulin or oral medications that can result in hypoglycemia should check their glucose before driving and at regular intervals when driving for periods of 1 hour or longer. Waiting to check glucose when symptoms of hypoglycemia arise is unsafe. Frequency of these intervals is individualized, so every 6 hours is incorrect and is too infrequent to be safe for most patients. It is safe for the patient to drive long periods of time as long as they regularly check their glucose levels.

55. D) Their LDL and triglycerides are both too high

The patient's triglycerides and LDL are above the desired ranges. Total cholesterol is desirable at lower than 200 mg/dL, with HDL at 40 or higher for men and 50 or higher for women, LDL lower than 70 for patients with diabetes, and triglycerides 150 or lower.

56. C) A high 2-hour level

The patient's 2-hour level is high, supporting a diagnosis of gestational diabetes. At least one or more values must exceed ranges for a positive diagnosis of gestational diabetes: over 92 mg/dL for fasting, over 180 mg/dL for 1 hour, over 153 mg/dL for 2 hours. Following current guidelines of a one-step method, further testing is not required to confirm diabetes, given the evidence of the patient's elevated glucose level at 2 hours. With the two-step method glucose tolerance test, two abnormal values are necessary to confirm diabetes.

57. A) Diabetic amyotrophy

The patient is likely experiencing diabetic amyotrophy. The symptoms of diabetic amyotrophy usually occur on one side of the body but can sometimes involve both sides. Autonomic neuropathy causes changes in digestion, bowel and bladder function, sexual response, and perspiration. Chronic inflammatory demyelinating polyneuropathy progresses slowly and causes symmetric weakness of muscles around the hips, shoulders, hands, and feet, but is unrelated to diabetes. Charcot–Marie–Tooth disease is a hereditary disorder that has similar presentation but is not commonly concurrent with diabetes.

58. C) Potassium

When a person in diabetic ketoacidosis is given insulin, the insulin drives potassium from the plasma into the cells, and the extracellular potassium is lost in urine from osmotic changes. These fluctuations cause low potassium or hypokalemia and require supplemental potassium to correct the electrolyte balance. Sodium, chloride, and phosphorus are not typically administered with insulin to a patient hospitalized with diabetic ketoacidosis.

59. C) The pain medication should not be taken within 2 hours of pramlintide

Pain medication should not be taken within 2 hours of pramlintide because pramlintide slows gastric emptying and therefore slows the absorption of oral medications. It is not necessary to switch from pramlintide to acarbose even though pramlintide cannot be taken simultaneously with pain medication. It is not necessary to increase the pramlintide dosage; timing is more important.

60. B) Low-fat diet
A low-fat diet would be appropriate for this patient. The patient's testing indicates gastroparesis, which can be aggravated by high-fat foods. A diet high in fiber is contraindicated because it can slow digestion even more. A gluten-free diet would be recommended for a positive test for celiac disease but is not relevant to this patient. A lactose-free diet is not relevant to gastric motility but rather to maldigestion of the milk sugar lactose.

61. D) Mononeuropathy
Mononeuropathy is the sudden onset of acute localized pain due to vascular obstruction. It tends to resolve spontaneously. Charcot joint refers to a neuropathic disorder that is most common as localized pain in the foot from collapsing bones. Entrapment syndrome is progressive and usually does not resolve spontaneously. Carpal tunnel syndrome is an example of entrapment syndrome. Diabetic amyotrophy causes weakness and wasting of muscles of the thighs, hips, buttocks, and legs.

62. B) "I have no appetite and I've lost 10 lb this month."
Reduced appetite and weight loss may indicate depression. Depression usually causes a lack of energy and fatigue, a loss of interest in hobbies and socialization, and feelings of hopelessness about the future. Feeling tired at times, setting goals such as working on hobbies, and positive thinking do not indicate feelings of hopelessness or loss of interest in activities that would cause the educator to consult a mental health professional.

63. C) Using a conversation map about taking medications
The patient demonstrates a need for active and sharing learning. A conversation map would be an effective way for the patient to actively learn while sharing relevant information and being interactive. A video or book would be appropriate if the patient showed a more passive learning style. Food models only enhance the learning experience and would not be as engaging for this patient.

64. D) "Readings will not reflect any rapid changes in glucose levels."
The educator should tell the patient that readings will not reflect any rapid changes in glucose because of the nature of changes in blood circulation of the fingers versus the arm. This indicates that in times of rapidly changing glucose levels, such as in hypoglycemia, after eating, or after exercise, alternate meters may lead to a delay or overtreatment of glucose levels. Alternate meters are accurate, but at a steady state, such as during fasting. Due to these limitations, alternate meters are not meant to be used in an emergency or as a comparison.

65. D) The DASH diet emphasizes sodium restriction

The DASH diet emphasizes a focus on sodium restriction for hypertension control more than the Mediterranean diet does. Both diets emphasize a plant-based meal pattern. The DASH diet does not limit but encourages two to three servings of low-fat dairy per day. Both diets allow meat, but the DASH diet emphasizes a reduction in saturated fats while the Mediterranean diet includes poultry in moderation and red meat only occasionally.

66. B) Be willing to listen and focus on basic skills and concepts

The educator should be willing to listen and focus on basic skills and concepts. Trying to distract the patient will not work and could result in the patient not returning for follow-up meetings. Trying to get the patient to open up about their feelings in a group education setting is most likely to be effective only during the depression phase of grief. Recommending an antidepressant is not appropriate for a diabetes educator unless they are also a mental health professional with prescribing authority.

67. C) Three

There are three carbohydrate choices in two servings of cookies. One carbohydrate choice, or serving, contains about 15 g of carbohydrates. Two carbohydrate choices contain about 30 g, and three carbohydrate choices contain 45 g of carbohydrate. Two servings of the cookies have 44 g of carbohydrate, which roughly equates to three carbohydrate choices.

68. A) The patient is gaining an appropriate amount of weight

The patient is gaining an appropriate amount of weight. A patient with a prepregnancy body mass index of 30+ should strive for 11 to 20 lb of weight gain throughout pregnancy. The current weight with a goal of 1/2 lb of weight gain for each additional week would put the patient on track to stay in the normal range. Gaining an additional 15 lb would be over the recommended total weight gain for this patient. Pregnant patients who have body mass indexes of 18.6 to 24.9 should aim to gain at a rate of 1 lb a week.

69. C) ACE inhibitors and ARBs reduce the risk of progressive kidney disease

ACE inhibitors and ARBs reduce the risk of progressive kidney disease. All of the classes of medication are likely safe for this patient, but only ACE inhibitors and ARBs reduce the risk of progressive kidney disease and decrease blood pressure. Raising blood glucose, increasing the risk of infection, and promoting weight loss are not the main concerns with other hypertension medications for patients with diabetes.

70. D) "Ask your child what is helpful for you to do."

It is best if the parents ask their child what is helpful for them to do. The parents' role during the teenage years is to be a support, yet monitor for signs of poor coping. The parents should ask the same question every so often because their child's needs might change throughout time. This respects their child's autonomy. Reassurance and positive reinforcement are more appropriate for a child of early elementary school age and are designed to enhance regimen compliance. Setting limits is a developmental goal for parents raising a toddler who may just be beginning to demonstrate interest in care participation but still requires parental choices and assistance. Assisting in regular glucose monitoring may be appropriate up to early elementary school age when parents should still be involved with self-care tasks.

71. A) Three-point profile

The three-point profile emphasizes a pattern to check fasting in the morning and then before and 2 hours after the largest meal. This pattern would be effective in providing feedback to the patient about the impact their largest meal has on their glucose control. Staggered and meal-based profiles emphasize a patterned variance and require two checks a day before and after different meals. Those patterns may not be as effective in feedback as the three-point profile. A five-point profile requires checking up to five times a day, which is more demanding and is unnecessary for this patient.

72. A) Endocrinologist for symptoms of Graves' disease

The patient should be referred to an endocrinologist because the patient has symptoms of Graves' disease, an autoimmune disease that is common in people with type 1 diabetes. A person with an eating disorder would not report an increased appetite. Symptoms of multiple sclerosis include paralysis, vertigo, incontinence or urinary retention, muscle spasticity and incoordination, and tremors. Symptoms of kidney failure include reduced urine output, swelling of the lower extremities, shortness of breath, drowsiness and confusion, nausea, and chest pain.

73. C) Norepinephrine

Norepinephrine reduces muscle uptake of glucose during exercise. Growth hormone and cortisol increase lipolysis and provide an increased supply of glycerol and amino acids to the liver. Glucagon stimulates glycogenolysis and gluconeogenesis.

74. B) Numeracy

The patient's ability to measure and evaluate carbohydrates is most likely lacking, which means they are likely lacking in numeracy. The patient does not specifically demonstrate lack of general literacy or inability to read. Document literacy would imply being able to apply a solution to an experienced health problem, such as following instructions when glucose is over 300. Prose literacy is the demonstration of following medical instructions such as those for administrating glucagon.

75. A) The participant will demonstrate the ability to safely and accurately monitor their blood glucose

"The participant will demonstrate the ability to safely and accurately monitor their blood glucose" is an example of a behavioral objective. A behavioral objective describes what the participant will be able to do after attending the program; it must be something that is observable and measurable. Verbs such as "appreciate," "believe," "know," "learn," "think," or "understand" are not written as measurable or observable so they are not as appropriate and should not be used when writing a behavioral objective.

76. A) Schedule interpreter services to be available for the session

Scheduling interpreter services to be available for the session would be an appropriate first step in preparing for a hearing-impaired individual. A video may be a useful tool but is not essential and does not allow for interaction. A white board can be a useful tool, but other visual tools such as props and handouts can be just as helpful. A family member may want to be present but is not qualified to assist in education; relying on untrained family members could lead to miscommunications or compromise patient privacy.

77. A) Review information on target goals and the safety of medications

The diabetes educator should review information on target goals and the safety of the medications. At this initial assessment, it would be most appropriate to review basic information. Providing encouragement to achieve the goal of becoming a great-grandparent is not appropriate, because meeting this goal is not within the patient's control. Documentation and referral would overlook the need to provide information and the need to address inconsistencies in beliefs and actual subjective information (A1C and blood pressure). Further reinforcing the patient's behavior will not be beneficial in moving this patient toward a more complete approach to treatment, including likely needed medications.

78. A) Metformin and basal insulin

An appropriate initial therapy is a combination of metformin and basal insulin. Combination injectable therapy should be considered when patients present with A1C levels >10%. A basal bolus would not be considered unless there is no improvement in the A1C. The combination of metformin with lifestyle changes would not be effective as an initial step. Adding a GLP-1 with basal insulin is more often recommended after treatment when metformin and basal insulin do not lead to improvement in A1C.

79. C) Suggest private spaces

Suggesting private spaces within the office is an appropriate follow-up solution for this patient. At this time, the patient is demonstrating inconvenience as a primary barrier. Many patients may not want to test their glucose levels in an open environment. Empty private rooms or the restroom may be more convenient. Reminder aids would help with cognitive-associated barriers. Time constraints and health literacy would require a review of necessary skills. The patient is not emotional, so acknowledging feelings would probably not yield any progress toward a solution.

80. C) Is on erythropoietin therapy

Testing for diabetes or prediabetes should be considered for all patients with a BMI of 25 or greater (BMI of 23 or greater in patients of Asian heritage) and one or more risk factors for diabetes. Polycystic ovary syndrome is a risk factor for diabetes. Pregnancy, recent blood transfusion, and receiving erythropoietin therapy increase red blood cell turnover, which ultimately affects the accuracy of an A1C test. Therefore, these situations would not be considered a reason to perform this test.

81. C) Measure the pressure several times 1 minute apart, and record the results

The patient should take measurements several times 1 minute apart and record the results. Checking blood pressure after resting and sitting quietly is better than after exercise. Cuffs should be carefully measured to arm circumference and not fit too snugly; this could lead to false high readings. Most pharmacy and public blood pressure machines should not be trusted since they are often not well maintained.

82. C) Decrease in production of incretin hormones that promote insulin production after eating

Patients with type 2 diabetes often have decreased production of incretin hormones caused by defective insulin secretions due to inflammation, metabolic stress, and genetic factors. Therefore, patients with metabolic stress syndrome will be affected, triggering hyperglycemic incidence. Decreased production of incretin hormones lowers insulin secretion after meals, leading to high levels of glucose in the blood. Other factors affecting the body in this manner include increased hepatic glucose production, decreased peripheral muscle uptake of glucose, and increased kidney reabsorption of glucose.

83. B) Refer to the emergency department to begin intravenous fluid replacement

Profound hyperglycemia with glucose levels above 800 mg/dL, mild abdominal pain with nausea and vomiting, lack of fever, and normal-smelling breath are all characteristic of hyperosmolar hyperglycemic syndrome (HHS). HHS is a medical emergency that leads to severe dehydration and requires fluid replacement. Insulin should not be started until the potassium level is known; it would be tested after fluid replacement has started. Obtaining an A1C level is not a priority, although one should be obtained during the hospitalization to determine appropriate outpatient therapy. Testing for zinc transporter antibodies, used to differentiate types of diabetes, is also not a priority because the patient likely has type 2 diabetes.

84. C) Obtain charts to review documentation of chosen behavior data

The next step is to obtain charts to review documentation of chosen behavior data. Doing so provides data for further consideration of possible solutions. Calling patients, revising the documentation, and conducting an in-service session are all solution steps that would occur before analyzing the problem.

85. D) Remain elevated and require further monitoring to determine therapy

Abnormal blood glucose levels in the first trimester of pregnancy suggest a diagnosis of type 2 diabetes or prediabetes, as opposed to gestational diabetes, so the patient's blood sugar level will likely remain elevated after delivery. However, further monitoring is necessary to determine therapy. Patients with preexisting type 2 diabetes or prediabetes have higher than normal blood glucose levels, and therefore blood glucose will not return to a normal reading without treatment. The patient's insulin resistance will decline after delivery, so glucose levels will not suddenly increase. There are many medications available to treat type 2 diabetes that may work for the patient but are contraindicated during pregnancy; therefore, the same therapy needed during pregnancy may not be appropriate.

86. A) Decrease the dose of long-acting insulin to 24 units before bed

The fasting blood glucose level is related to the dose of long- or intermediate-acting insulin. This patient's dose of long-acting insulin needs to be adjusted to increase fasting glucose levels, which are below the recommended range. Any change in insulin doses should be made every 2 to 3 days in 10% to 20% increments. Decreasing the dose of long-acting insulin to 20 units is not appropriate because this is more than a 20% decrease and would likely lead to fasting blood glucose levels above the target. Splitting the dose of long-acting insulin into 15 units in the morning and 15 units before bed is not appropriate because it does not reduce the total dose of long-acting insulin. Changing the carbohydrate ratio to 1 to 8 is not advised because the patient's premeal blood glucose levels are mostly within the recommended range.

87. D) Work with the patient to set realistic blood sugar goals initially post discharge

The patient has been nonadherent to wearing their pump for at least 2 weeks. If aggressive blood sugar targets are sought upon discharge, it may set the patient up for failure. Additionally, the patient may fear weight gain with the use of additional insulin, and therefore an open discussion about this possibility is necessary. Tightened blood sugar goals can be targeted once the patient begins to wear the insulin pump regularly and begins to achieve goals set at discharge. Normalizing blood glucose rapidly can cause the patient to have symptoms of hypoglycemia and thus make them less adherent to goals. Keeping the insulin pump attached consistently will assist in achieving fewer instances of hyperglycemia and more stabilized overall blood glucose levels.

88. B) Learn how to quantify carbohydrate intake to match mealtime insulin doses

The best nutrition strategy for insulin in patients with type 1 and type 2 diabetes involves portion control, high-fiber carbohydrate options, and leaner protein options. Learning carbohydrate counting to match insulin intake is the best strategy for postprandial glucose readings. Eating meals based on a pattern or schedule helps to facilitate stabilization of blood sugars and prevents insulin stacking. Taking insulin 15 minutes before a meal, rather than postprandial, allows the insulin to absorb into the bloodstream simultaneously with the carbohydrate consumption. Eating an undefined amount of carbohydrates can promote hyperglycemia and inhibit optimal insulin absorption and timing.

89. C) Age 35 years

Screening for all asymptomatic adults should begin at age 35 years regardless of other risk factors. Screening for prediabetes is indicated for individuals with a BMI of $\geq$25 kg/m^2 ($\geq$23 kg/m^2 in those of Asian heritage), triglyceride levels $\geq$250 mg/dL, and BP $\geq$140/90.

90. B) Consume 30 to 60 g of carbohydrates prior to practice

Increasing carbohydrate intake by 30 to 60 g prior to practice (or 0.5–1.0 g/kg/hr of exercise) would be an acceptable first step in resolving the patient's hypoglycemic episodes. Although lowering basal insulin may be appropriate, lowering by 60% is excessive and likely would not allow the patient to maintain target glucose levels. Athletic activities provide excellent physical, mental, and social benefits and do not need to be discontinued or skipped unless the patient is unable to maintain safe glucose levels by implementing other strategies. If the patient's blood glucose levels are not at goal prior to exercise, it is possible to make insulin or dietary adjustments rather than skip practice.

91. C) Offer the option of a telemedicine visit

Telemedicine is useful for reaching patients who are unable to attend or have difficulty attending in-person appointments. It has been shown to be effective at reducing A1C in patients with type 2 diabetes. Labeling the patient as noncompliant to their provider does not facilitate a positive relationship between the provider, educator, and patient and does not serve to assist the patient in obtaining education. Refusing to see the patient severs the patient-educator relationship that the patient is trying to establish. Considering that the patient is already aware of and interested in an appointment, a letter about the service would be redundant.

92. B) Intensifying the medication regimen

One goal of the care team is to avoid therapeutic inertia in the population of diabetes patients. Considering that the patient has had 6 months with their new medication and it has not been effective, it is an appropriate time to intensify therapy. Continuing the current regimen, following up in 3 months, and allowing the patient additional time will only contribute to therapeutic inertia by keeping the patient not at goal with no specific intervention that will improve glycemic control.

93. C) Begin by selecting one problem to be discussed and have everyone state the problem clearly, using "I" statements

Adolescent patients with type 1 diabetes can present unique challenges to disease management when they assert control over their disease and feel that their parents are restrictive to their independence. When issues with type 1 diabetes arise, the educator must understand how to discuss these issues with the patient and their family. Defining one problem between family members allows for the flow of the conversation to be focused on differences in the way people view the importance of the issue, not on the patient being "the problem." Discussing every issue with the family is not constructive, and priorities can get lost in the conversation. Patients should use "I" statements, but the educator must avoid allowing accusations in the discussion. Identifying roles is important to knowing the expectations of each family member, but it is not necessary to choose a primary communicator.

94. A) Corticosteroid drug use

Diabetes can be drug induced. The most frequent cause of drug-induced diabetes is corticosteroid use. While infection, excessive carbohydrate intake, and inadequate insulin dosage may lead to increased blood glucose levels, the most frequent cause is overuse of corticosteroids.

95. D) Set up an education session for general medicine floor providers and nurses

According to the American Diabetes Association Standards of Care, the appropriate glycemic target for a hospitalized patient with diabetes on insulin who is not critically ill is 140 to 180 mg/dL. The staff on the unit must be educated about this standard so they can make a change in their practice. While it is true that there are different goals for different types of patients, explaining this to the patient does not address the issue. The stated goal was not appropriate for the circumstances. An apology may help to mend the patient's dissatisfaction, but it does not work to correct the problem. Even though this happened in an inpatient setting, the educator has a responsibility to identify errors, manage risks, and mentor staff as necessary to comply with practice standards and advocate for patient safety.

96. D) Correlation of high doses of acetylsalicylic acid (aspirin) to hypoglycemia

Large doses of salicylates, including acetylsalicylic acid (aspirin), can cause decreases in blood glucose levels. There is no known risk of taking appropriate doses of simvastatin (Zocor) and aspirin together. Injury and stress can affect blood glucose levels, often by increasing them; however, the educational priority is to address and rectify the patient's hypoglycemic episodes.

97. C) Add empagliflozin (Jardiance)

Sodium-glucose co-transporter 2 (SGLT2) inhibitors such as empagliflozin have been shown to slow chronic kidney disease (CKD) progression and are indicated for all patients with diabetes and CKD stage 3 or higher. An elevated A1C and decrease in eGFR indicate the need for a change in regimen. An increase in metformin is not appropriate due to the decrease in kidney function. Increasing insulin glargine (Lantus) is not appropriate due to the fasting blood glucose being on the low end of the target goal.

98. B) Discuss the patient's physical abilities and interests and help them set realistic goals following this assessment

Physical activity for both type 1 and type 2 diabetes can improve insulin sensitivity, help with weight control, reduce cardiovascular outcomes, and promote a sense of well-being. Exercise should be an integral part of the treatment plan for all patients with diabetes. Meeting the patient at their level of physical activity and capability is important for adherence to their goals. A recommendation of 150 minutes of exercise every week with 2 days of resistance training is a framework to work up to for exercise, but it may not be feasible for all patients, particularly when they are just starting. Likewise, facilitating high-intensity interval training may be beyond the patient's capabilities when starting a new exercise regimen. Instructing a patient to achieve goals beyond their desire or ability will lead to the patient being discouraged and therefore unsuccessful in reaching and maintaining realistic health goals.

99. B) Advise patient to continue the current plan as long as normal blood glucose levels are maintained

As long as the patient is maintaining normal blood glucose levels with the current medication regimen, there is no need to modify it. There are no data to suggest long-acting insulin is safer for this patient, whose diabetes is currently well controlled. There have been no studies showing insulin crossing into the placenta or increasing risk during pregnancy. Initiating an insulin pump therapy routine would be best as an option post pregnancy, not during pregnancy.

100. D) GAD antibodies, anti-islet cell antibodies, fasting insulin, non-fasting C-peptide levels, TSH, and antithyroid antibodies

The provider suspects that the patient has maturity-onset diabetes of the young (MODY). Types of diabetes other than type 1 and type 2 can be caused by genetic defects in insulin action, exocrine pancreatic diseases, and genetic defects in B cell function; many labs are required to make a differential diagnosis. A repeat postprandial glucose would not be necessary because it was elevated previously. A nonfasting C-peptide would assist in the diagnosis because it demonstrates the capability of insulin secretion after eating, but by itself it is not definitive. Hemoglobin will not assist in a diagnosis. TSH and antithyroid antibodies are key factors in autoimmune disorders and can accompany a type 1 diagnosis. Another A1C would not be necessary because these do not vary considerably within a 3-month window.

101. C) Glucose level at the time of testing

Not testing when the glucose level is high is the best explanation for why the A1C does not match the glucose log. The time of the test is also important, but this information is revealed in the records and contributes to the A1C level. The brand of testing strips used and the site where the specimen was taken are not factors in an A1C mismatch.

102. A) Patient illness

Patient illness is a factor that can impact glucose levels and contribute to the overall picture and the A1C level. Weather and temperature shifts can elicit small changes in glucose levels, but not enough change for additional records to be kept. Although a life change can cause stress that may affect glucose levels, a new job in and of itself would not require additional glucose records unless the patient reported heightened stress.

103. B) Has a urinary tract infection with or without symptoms

Any kind of infection that causes an increase in glucose levels can be a cause of HHS. A high-carbohydrate or high-protein meal will likely not contribute to HHS. HHS is a complication seen more frequently in older adults, not young adults.

104. C) Refer patient to a psychologist, counselor, psychiatrist, or social worker

A referral to a psychologist, counselor, psychiatrist, or social worker is appropriate after an affirmation of depression is expressed by a patient. Telling the patient that things will be fine or that their depression is hormonal is dismissive of the patient's feelings. Relating a story about a family member with diabetes is also dismissive and would not be an appropriate response.

105. C) Identify the problem

Identifying the problem is the first step in goal setting, followed by setting the goal, brainstorming ways to accomplish the goal, and evaluating the goal. The patient should discuss potential solutions with their healthcare team rather than determine solutions entirely on their own. Having patients set an action plan with short-term goals is more realistic, and the clinician can easily follow up the action plan. Long-term goals can be established once the short-term goals have become habit. Setting an action plan and determining the length of time before reevaluation of the goal is the final step. Imagining an ideal scenario will not be effective when the goal is to determine realistic solutions for a defined problem.

106. D) Diabetes

Diabetes is diagnosed by either classic symptoms of hyperglycemia and a random plasma glucose of 200 or greater or two abnormal screening tests, either from the same sample or in two separate test samples. This patient has diabetes because they have two abnormal screening tests: two A1C results of 6.5 or greater. Although this patient's FPG is consistent with prediabetes, their diagnosis is made based on the confirmatory screening test, which in this case is a repeat A1C. Abnormal glucose tolerance, or the inability to maintain normal glucose levels following oral administration of glucose, does not apply to this patient because A1C and FPG tests do not involve glucose administration. Euglycemia, or normal glucose in the blood, is not this patient's diagnosis because the patient's A1C results and FPG are above the normal range.

107. C) Negotiate a testing strategy that is based on what the patient is willing to do

The patient is most likely to be motivated by discussion and negotiation that is based on what the patient is willing to do. Having someone else test the patient's glucose level would not be motivating for the patient; involving a caregiver can be appropriate but would require the patient to willingly agree. Having the patient test after foods they like, such as soda or candy, might demonstrate to them how high their sugars go and motivate them to change their behavior; having them test after foods they dislike would not supply the same motivation. Testing while feeling "funny" or unwell can be insightful to patients, especially if they find that they are hypoglycemic or hyperglycemic during these times. Testing while feeling well would not have the same impact.

108. B) Instruct the patient in lifestyle changes and recommend that the provider start the patient on a medication for blood pressure
Neglecting to treat hypertension or waiting for a week or more to assess blood pressure would be unsafe for a patient with uncontrolled hypertension. The patient's hypertension should be treated immediately with initiation and timely titration of a pharmacologic agent such as an angiotensin-converting enzyme (ACE) inhibitor, an angiotensin II receptor blocker (ARB), a thiazide-like diuretic, or a calcium channel blocker. These are all appropriate medication choices for a patient with diabetes.

109. D) Timing of insulin use
An important factor to consider when evaluating the cause of hypoglycemia is the timing of insulin use by the patient. The patient's emotional condition would not be a contributing factor to hypoglycemia, but a change in emotional condition can be a symptom of a hypoglycemic episode. The place the testing was done and any assistance the patient received with testing would not be factors of significance when evaluating the cause of hypoglycemia.

110. D) Peripheral neuropathy
Peripheral neuropathy is a long-term complication exacerbated by uncontrolled glucose levels, but it is not a condition directly caused by diabetes. HHS, DKA, and hypoglycemia are all considered acute complications of either uncontrolled diabetes or of a misuse of hypoglycemic agents.

111. A) National Diabetes Prevention Program
The National Diabetes Prevention Program is a program offered to patients with prediabetes through the Diabetes Prevention Recognition Program. This would be the best resource for a patient with prediabetes to learn more about the condition. Only patients already diagnosed with diabetes are eligible for the Living with Diabetes Educational series. The American Heart Association is not oriented only to diabetes and thus would not be the best resource for a patient with prediabetes. The U.S. Department of Agriculture offers the MyPlate initiative, which offers general nutrition information and is not specifically focused on prediabetes or diabetes.

112. D) How optimistic are you about your diagnosis?

Asking the patient to rate their optimism would not be helpful or appropriate. Asking the patient how they learn best can offer insight when determining how to help the patient retain knowledge. Understanding the patient's education level can suggest ways that simple or complex information should be presented. Knowing if a patient is forgetful can offer the educator cues on how to assist the patient in remembering.

113. A) Rapid-acting insulin has a faster absorption at 15 minutes, making it more conducive to improved glucose levels postprandial

Rapid-acting insulin has an onset of 15 minutes, making bolusing before meals a much easier task than with regular insulin, which can take between 0.5 and 1 hour for onset. This is important for the patient's postprandial glucose levels and improves compliance with taking insulin as well, because it will be more effective. The main advantage of rapid-acting insulin is not financial; regular insulin is cheaper but is inferior in terms of onset and duration.

114. B) During the assessment

Questions and concerns identified by the patient should be addressed at the beginning of the education process, during the assessment step. This helps tailor the education to the patient's individualized needs and increases the effectiveness of the education. Waiting until the middle or the end of the program would not allow the diabetes educator to individualize the education. The outcome evaluation addresses patient and programmatic outcomes, not the patient's concerns and questions.

115. D) Ask the parents to get more involved with the patient's glucose testing

Asking the parents to be more involved will only exacerbate tensions about the patient's lack of management. Asking the patient about their perception of their parents' involvement and then how much the patient is involved in their own care will highlight the ineffective communication between them. This will open the door for negotiation within the family and can allow the parents more involvement in managing the patient's diabetes.

116. D) "I will not worry because tracking my glucose and my insulin dosing is not important."

The patient should be taught the importance of tracking glucose and insulin dosing and that it can be managed effectively without a continuous glucose monitor. Available technology allows patients to upload their glucose levels via computer or smart device. Bolus calculators also exist for dosing insulin. However, it is important to assess what the patient can afford, what they will be able to learn, and what their insurance will authorize before choosing the appropriate tool for testing.

117. C) Does not use insulin-to-carbohydrate ratios

The patient who does not use insulin-to-carbohydrate ratios is limited in their understanding of carbohydrate counting and would have to dose insulin based on units rather than carbohydrates. A patient planning a pregnancy, a patient with frequent low blood glucose levels, and a patient who has an erratic schedule would all be appropriate candidates for insulin pump therapy.

118. B) Video or internet-based program

Video or internet-based programs are not an effective follow-up method for patients because they likely include no interaction or opportunity to ask personal questions or share concerns. While there are some limitations, a telephone call with a diabetes educator and a virtual appointment with a registered dietitian nutritionist would be more effective and allow the patient and the diabetes educator to ask questions and problem solve together. An in-person shared medical appointment would be effective, would allow the patient to easily bring food records and blood glucose logs, and would provide additional support.

119. C) Connected insulin pen

A connected insulin pen would best match the patient's needs and preferences because it can be programmed to calculate insulin doses based on entered blood sugar values, planned carbohydrate intake, and IOB, similar to an insulin pump but without anything attached to the body. An implanted sensor cannot be programed to calculate doses and does not keep track of IOB. It also requires the patient to wear a removable smart transmitter to see their glucose data. Intermittent CGM also cannot be programmed to calculate doses and does not keep track of IOB. However, it may be appropriate for a patient who would benefit from CGM but does not want to wear a device all the time. Tubeless insulin pumps can be programmed to calculate doses and keep track of IOB and do not contain tubing. However, tubeless insulin pump therapy requires the patient to wear a pod containing a cannula and insulin attached directly to their body.

120. B) Onset (hours): <0.5–1; peak: dual; effective duration (hours): 10–16

70% NPH, 30% regular insulin has an onset of 0.5 to 1 hour, a dual peak (when the regular insulin peaks and then the NPH insulin peaks) with a duration of 10 to 16 hours.

121. B) Basal insulin accounts for 40% to 60% of the total daily insulin, and the bolus should account for the remaining percentage (divided into three doses for meals)

Typically, basal insulin should account for 40% to 60% of the total daily insulin, and the remainder amount would be administered as bolus doses, divided based on meal composition and content. A patient may have a lower bolus amount if they are eating a lower-carbohydrate diet, but generally this is a starting point for patients who are newly diagnosed and starting insulin.

122. C) Onset (hours): <0.01–0.05; peak: 0.12–0.15 (hours); effective duration (hours): 3

Inhaled insulin has a rapid absorption at 0.01 to 0.05 (hours), peaks at 0.12 to 0.15 (hours), and has a duration of 3 hours.

123. D) "How important is checking your blood glucose levels to you?"

To increase effectiveness of disease management, it is important to integrate emotional components into questions and avoid asking patients "yes or no" questions. Asking patients "why" questions can place them on the defensive instead of providing support. Asking open-ended questions can assist the patient to incorporate new behaviors more readily.

124. B) 3 to 5 hours is a normal amount of time to see a blood sugar correction

It takes 3 to 5 hours to see a correction for hyperglycemia return to the baseline due to the duration of action of rapid- and short-acting insulin. A decreased correction factor would mean that more insulin would be delivered to correct blood sugar and would likely result in hypoglycemia. Hyperglycemia cannot always be prevented in patients with type 1 diabetes because there are multiple factors that impact glucose levels. The carbohydrate ratio is not a consideration when addressing correction factor.

125. A) 50 mg/dL
An increase in blood glucose of more than 50 mg/dL after meals triggers reactive oxidative stress, which has been implicated in both microvascular and macrovascular complications of diabetes. An increase of more than 20 mg/dL after meals represents a normal fluctuation of glucose. Increases of more than 80 mg/dL or more than 100 mg/dL are above the threshold for triggering reactive oxidative stress.

126. B) 5 years after their diagnosis
Adults with newly diagnosed type 1 diabetes should be referred to ophthalmology for an initial dilation and comprehensive eye examination 5 years after the onset of diabetes. Timely diagnosis of diabetic retinopathy allows intervention that may prevent vision loss in patients who are asymptomatic despite diabetic eye disease. Referrals at the time of diagnosis, within 2 years of diagnosis if glycemia is well controlled, and 1 year after diagnosis would be too soon; retinopathy is estimated to take at least 5 years to develop after the onset of hyperglycemia.

127. C) 11 to 12 years
Transition planning should begin at 11 to 12 years of age for most pediatric patients to allow time for the patient to develop necessary skills. At this first stage of planning, the healthcare provider, the patient, and the family should review the expected age of transfer, the patient's responsibilities for preparing for transition, the parental responsibilities, and the healthcare team member's responsibilities. Age 18 to 21 is when the final step occurs and the patient either transfers to an adult provider or remains under the care of a pediatric provider under an adult care model. Age 14 is when the second step occurs and a formalized and individualized transition plan is developed. Age 15 to 17 is when the third step occurs and the patient, the family, and the healthcare team review the plan, assess achieved goals, and problem-solve barriers to remaining goals.

128. D) At diagnosis, annually and/or when the patient does not meet treatment targets, when factors develop that influence self-management, and when transitions in life and care occur

The need for DSMES should be evaluated by the healthcare team members, with referrals made as needed, at diagnosis, annually and/or when the patient does not meet treatment targets, when complicating factors (health conditions, physical limitations, emotional factors, or basic living needs) develop that influence self-management, and when transitions in life and care occur, according to the 2022 American Diabetes Association (ADA) Standards of Medical Care in Diabetes. Evaluating the need for DSMES when the A1C is >9%, 6 months after the patient has completed a DSME program, when insulin therapy is initiated, when the patient requests DSMES, and when complications of diabetes develop are not specific times recommended in the 2022 ADA Standards of Medical Care in Diabetes, although they may coincide with some of the critical time points.

129. D) Contact the patient to obtain glucose data and adjust doses in between visits

The patient should be contacted to discuss glucose data and adjust doses in between visits. Pregnancy is timely and it is important to adjust insulin at frequent intervals, including when insulin is started and when targets are not being met. Using guidelines based on weight and gestational age to determine insulin doses is an effective way to initiate insulin, but these doses will need to be adjusted to reach glycemic targets. Teaching the patient to make self-adjustments based on glucose data, food intake, and activity level is not a realistic goal for a patient with gestational diabetes who is new to insulin. The patient should be instructed to keep a glucose log and bring it to their appointments, but they will still require contact between appointments.

130. A) Biguanide and thiazolidinedione

The provider should prescribe a biguanide and a thiazolidinedione. It is important for providers to address self-management barriers and provide glycemic management that is patient centered. In this case, the patient has stated that cost and fear of hypoglycemia are barriers for them. Biguanides and thiazolidinediones are low-cost options that do not cause hypoglycemia. Second-generation sulfonylureas can cause hypoglycemia. Insulin is high in cost and can cause hypoglycemia. GLP-1 receptor agonists are also high in cost.

131. C) Reassess the goal with the patient and consider possible revisions
The diabetes educator and the patient should reassess the goal and consider possible revisions. Revisions to the goal should be self-directed, achievable, and realistic. Scheduling the patient for a follow-up in 6 months to allow more time to achieve the goal is inappropriate because the original goal is not realistic or achievable. Furthermore, longer-term follow-ups have been shown to be less effective than shorter-term follow-ups in facilitating behavioral change. Providing digital coaching and asking the patient how they will feel after they achieve a goal are effective strategies but only if the identified goal is achievable and realistic.

132. C) Decrease their long-acting insulin
The provider should recommend decreasing the long-acting insulin because the fasting blood sugars are below the fasting target of 80 to 130 mg/dL for patients taking insulin. The preprandial glucose values before breakfast are above the recommended range of 80 to 130 for most patients on insulin, but this may be due to overtreatment of their fasting blood sugars. The low fasting blood sugars should be addressed first, and then any values above the target can be addressed. The preprandial glucose values for lunch and dinner are within the recommended range. Increasing mealtime insulin with breakfast and decreasing long-acting insulin would not be appropriate because hypoglycemia should be addressed prior to addressing hyperglycemia. A high preprandial glucose value prior to dinner, not a high preprandial reading at breakfast, would be an indication to increase the mealtime insulin at lunch. The patient should not have breakfast earlier because low fasting blood sugars are indicative of too much long-acting insulin, which can cause hypoglycemia throughout the night as well as in the morning.

133. D) 48
Increased insulin sensitivity post physical exercise is lost in 48 hours, which is why recurrent exercise is important for diabetes prevention and management.

134. C) "Was the coffee black?"
Inquiring further about the coffee may provide insight into potential added carbohydrates, including creamer and sugar. One packet or teaspoon of sugar equals 3 to 4 g of carbohydrates, and one teaspoon of regular creamer equals 2 to 4 g of carbohydrates. Depending on the patient's use and servings of sugar and creamer, their total carbohydrate count for the meal may be significantly higher than realized and reported. Eating whole eggs versus egg whites would affect protein, fat, and calorie content. While wheat bread may include more fiber, it is unlikely that it would affect blood sugar as significantly as the potential added carbohydrates from sugar and creamer. Some apple varieties do contain higher levels of sugar, but it is unlikely that this would significantly affect the patient's blood glucose level when only one apple is eaten.

135. A) Assessment, diagnosis, intervention, monitoring, and evaluation (ADIME)

The current medical nutrition therapy and documentation is ADIME: assessment, diagnosis, intervention, monitoring, and evaluation. The SOAP note stands for subjective, objective, assessment, and plan. While it is widely used among many healthcare disciplines, the current documentation standard is ADIME. Nutrition assessment can be performed using the ABCD method, which stands for anthropometry, biochemistry, clinical, and diet. A PES statement is a component of the ADIME diagnosis and stands for problem, etiology, and signs/symptoms.

136. A) Eat half the banana at breakfast and save the other half for a snack

The patient's breakfast equals approximately 77 g of carbohydrates, which exceeds the patient's goal of 45 to 60 g per meal. Many newly diagnosed patients do not realize that one banana has 30 g of carbohydrates and often assume it has 15 g. Eating half of the banana at breakfast and saving the other half for a snack would keep the patient's breakfast at goal. The patient's lunch, dinner, and snack are within the range of 45 to 60 g of carbohydrates per meal or 0 to 15 g per snack.

137. A) Aim for weight loss of 15 to 20 lb

Treatment recommendations for patients with prediabetes would include lifestyle modification consisting of 5% to 10% weight loss and moderate-intensity exercise for approximately 30 minutes per day. A 15- to 20-lb weight loss for this patient would be appropriate at approximately 7% to 10% of total body weight. Elimination of carbohydrates from the diet is not necessary, realistic for most patients, or healthy. A recommendation of 45 to 60 minutes of moderate to intense exercise per day exceeds the recommendation and could possibly be unsafe for a patient just initiating exercise. While insulin may be necessary for this patient in the future, recommending insulin when/if their A1C increases does not help the patient with their current question and their desire to prevent diabetes.

138. B) Two slices from a medium pepperoni pizza, diet soda

The carbohydrate count for two slices of a medium pizza and a diet soda would fall within the carbohydrate goal of 45 to 60 g of carbohydrates per meal. The "open face" cold-cut sandwich meal would equal approximately 65 to 70 g of carbohydrates and would exceed the goal. The chicken caesar salad meal would equal approximately 20 g of carbohydrates and would not be sufficient. The burger and fries meal would equal more than 80 g of carbohydrates and would exceed goal.

139. B) Hypoxemia and high-dose vitamin C

Some glucose monitors are sensitive to oxygen available, and a patient with hypoxemia may receive false high blood glucose readings. Similarly, patients receiving high-dose vitamin C supplementation may also receive falsely elevated readings. There is no correlation between a patient being diagnosed with hyperthyroidism and receiving inaccurate blood glucose readings.

140. D) Fasting and 2 hours postprandially

With self-monitoring of blood glucose and pattern management, the blood glucose level is checked fasting and 2 hours postprandially. Checking blood glucose levels every 4 to 6 hours without regard for fasting or meal status would not provide helpful data. Fasting is an appropriate time to monitor, but before bedtime may not provide relevant data depending on when the patient's last meal was eaten. One hour postprandially would not give enough time for the full blood glucose effect of the patient's meal to be represented when checked.

141. A) Downloadable data reports

One of the benefits of a "smart pen" is downloadable data reports, including blood glucose readings, insulin doses, and dose reminders. A "smart pen" would not provide continuous glucose monitoring as an insulin pump would. Using an insulin pen would not change the patient's carbohydrate requirements or goals but should help the patient achieve better blood glucose control while following their plan. If the patient was prescribed basal insulin, the "smart pen" would not replace the basal insulin but would work in combination to keep blood glucose at goal.

142. C) Ineffective insulin and testing strips

Insulin that is expired or stored in extreme temperatures can become ineffective. Due to the patient's report of homelessness and a period of living in their car, it is likely that the insulin was exposed to extreme temperatures. Due to the large supply of insulin boxes the patient brought to clinic, it is possible that they are expired and that the patient has not refilled their prescriptions recently. Expired test strips can also provide incorrect and variable results. Food insecurity, inconsistent carbohydrate intake, inadequate physical activity, and weight gain can all contribute to elevated blood sugar levels; however, this information was not provided in the patient's report or assessment. Inadequate bolus insulin would result in elevated blood glucose levels; however, the diabetes educator verified that the patient had a correct understanding of their plan.

143. D) "Are you taking your bolus insulin before or after your meal?"

Clarifying if the patient is taking their bolus insulin before or after meals may provide an answer to their erratic blood sugar levels. A common self-management error is taking bolus insulin after meals due to variable amount of food, irregular schedule, and fear of administering excessive insulin. This reactive versus proactive use of insulin can lead to variable and/or elevated blood sugar readings as the patient's blood sugar has likely already spiked by the time they administer their bolus insulin. Initially questioning the patient on compliance related to insulin doses and carbohydrate intake will not help build rapport with a patient who has already expressed compliance and is struggling with the desire to manage their diabetes independently. The patient's physical activity level can definitely impact their blood glucose levels but would likely not be the biggest contributing factor to their recent elevated and variable readings.

144. C) Evening alcohol intake

Drinking alcohol can put the patient at risk for delayed hypoglycemia, especially if they are taking insulin. Inadequate carbohydrate intake at dinner would put the patient at risk for a hypoglycemic episode; however, it would likely occur sooner after the meal than as a delayed response in the middle of the night. Some patients benefit from a small carbohydrate snack in the evening, but ideally their glucose management should not be so dependent on a snack to maintain safe levels. Vigorous exercise can cause sudden or delayed hypoglycemia; however, low-intensity exercise with a short duration would not be the most likely cause of this patient's delayed hypoglycemia.

145. A) Take an additional blood glucose reading at 3:00 a.m.

If there is a pattern of elevated fasting glucose levels, an appropriate next step would be to ask the patient to take an additional blood glucose reading at 3:00 a.m. at least once or twice a week to help determine the cause. There are multiple potential reasons for elevated fasting glucose levels, including overnight hypoglycemic episodes, insufficient insulin, and dawn phenomenon. Reducing dinner carbohydrates is not the best way to determine the reason for the elevated fasting readings and could be unhelpful if the patient is having overnight hypoglycemia. While it is possible that alcohol consumption may cause delayed hypoglycemia, it is unknown if the patient is consuming alcohol in the evening. Initiating exercise may be a positive self-management strategy for this patient but would not give the diabetes educator additional information on the root cause of the elevated fasting glucose level. Increasing exercise would be a reactive recommendation.

146. D) Continuous glucose monitor (CGM)

A CGM would reduce or eliminate the need for fingers sticks and would also provide downloadable data that the diabetes educator and the patient's child could use to evaluate efficacy and compliance of the patient's diabetes care plan. An insulin "smart pen" may be helpful for providing insulin usage, but the patient would need either a CGM or to continue finger sticks to determine current blood sugar levels. An automatic blood glucose monitor is fairly new technology that eliminates the need for testing strips but would not help with the patient's pain levels. A smaller-gauge lancet may reduce the patient's pain level but may also result in difficulty obtaining a large enough blood sample and would not provide any data to the diabetes educator or the family member.

147. C) Refer the patient to a shared medical appointment

A shared medical appointment would be a great resource for this patient as it would provide them additional education and access to a collaborative team. The patient would likely receive services from a team of physicians, nurses, pharmacists, registered dietitian nutritionists, social workers, and/or behaviorists. Repeating the DSME class could be helpful, but this patient would better benefit from more personalized support at this time. An online diabetes class would likely not help the patient with their motivation or allow them to engage with anyone to receive individual care. Showing sympathy and providing reassurance is important when interacting with patients; however, the best approach would be to provide the patient with tangible ways to help them manage their diabetes.

148. B) Diabetes support group

A diabetes support group would be a great option for this patient to provide ongoing education, social support, motivation, and accountability. A service dog trained in diabetes care would be helpful for a patient struggling to manage their diabetes due to physical limitations, mobility, and recurrent hypoglycemia. However, this patient is struggling with motivation, not ability to manage their diabetes. Many patients find phone or computer tracking applications to be motivational; however, this patient would likely benefit from the social aspect of a support group because they mentioned feeling lonely and isolated from family. A meal delivery service may be helpful for consistent consumption of carbohydrates if the patient is able to select meals that are within their carbohydrate goal; however, a meal delivery service would not likely help the patient's motivation level related to tracking their blood glucose levels.

149. D) Work with the patient to determine a carbohydrate goal that the patient feels would be realistic for them

Nutrition therapy interventions and recommendations should be patient specific and must meet the patient's goals and lifestyle. The interventions will only be effective if the patient is willing to implement them. The patient is resistant to the RDN's recommendation, and working together to find a realistic goal that the patient agrees to would likely increase compliance and build rapport. Maintaining the original recommendation or requesting that the patient try the recommendation without attempting to work toward creating a mutually agreed-upon goal will most likely not result in improved glycemic control for this patient. If the patient consumes more carbohydrates than needed, it is possible they will need to have their medications adjusted; however, stating this could be perceived as threatening to the patient and will not help establish rapport.

150. D) Setting a goal of diabetes management interdependence

Interdependence is defined as the use of friends and family to help and support diabetes management. It is beneficial to discuss the goal of interdependence versus independence, especially in adolescents with diabetes. Many adolescents desire freedom to manage their diabetes independently; however, they should be encouraged to use the support and guidance of parents, family, and friends to help them achieve the goal of independence as they grow and mature. Some parents with generally responsible and intelligent children may encourage independence earlier than the adolescent is ready for; as managing diabetes, emotional health, school work, extracurriculars, and social life can become burdensome and overwhelming for adolescents. Problem-solving skills are an important aspect of diabetes management, especially with such an irregular schedule, but the priority topic during this conversation would be encouraging the patient to be receptive to parental support and for the parent to maintain an active supporting role. Diabetes care is important and is necessary to safely engage in many athletic activities, but there is no reason to assume the patient is not prioritizing their care or that their activities need to be reduced. Parents should play a supporting role in their adolescent's diabetes management that is specific to their child's age, maturity level, and cognitive level.

151. A) Refer patients for an outpatient diabetes educator consultation prior to and after treatment

The dentist referring patients to individualized outpatient education before and after treatment will best help the patients work through preparing, problem-solving, and achieving optimal blood glucose control, which will promote faster and safer recoveries. Mailing educational materials or providing a video is impersonal, does not provide any information about the patients' current blood sugar control, and does not allow the patients to ask questions. A referral to a DSME class may be helpful, but it is likely that many patients have already attended a class. DSME classes are often taught in a series over several weeks, which may not allow patients to receive the information they need before their dental treatment is needed.

152. B) Miscarried helping

Miscarried helping, also known as emotional overinvolvement, shows how the good intentions of others in supporting an individual with a chronic health condition can result in interpersonal conflict, poorer health behaviors, and poorer health outcomes. During this appointment, it appears that the patient is feeling blamed and not trusted, and the parents are exhibiting frustration with the patient's current blood glucose control. Interdependence is defined as the use of friends and family to help and support diabetes management. Active parental involvement would consist of appropriate and helpful participation in the patient's health and other aspects of life, including academics and athletics. Parental reinforcement is a parenting strategy that seeks to encourage and achieve desired behavior.

153. C) Registered dietitian nutritionist

Appropriate and adequate nutrition intake is crucial for a patient with CF and diabetes. Their increased metabolic requirements and need for a "matched insulin regimen" add another layer of complexity to their care plan. Patients with CF also have specific dietary requirements of high-calorie, high-fat, and high-sodium foods, with about 15% to 20% of the diet consisting of protein. An exercise physiologist and clinical psychologist may also be a recommended part of the patient's care team but would not play as critical of a role in affecting the patient's outcomes. Some cancers are more prevalent in patients with CF, but an oncologist is not a primary member of the healthcare team.

154. B) 13 to 18
The USDPP's goal for patients in the lifestyle change group was to lose 5% to 7% of total body weight and to exercise for at least 150 minutes per week. The study found that patients who lost and sustained approximately 5% weight loss had a 58% decreased risk of developing type 2 diabetes. Thirteen to 18 lb is 5% to 7% of the patient's current body weight, which would meet the USDPP's goal. A 5- to 10-lb weight loss would be 2% to 4% weight loss, 20 to 25 lb would be 8% to 10%, and 23 to 30 lb would be 9% to 12%.

155. D) U.S. Diabetes Prevention Program (USDPP)
The USDPP was the largest of the six major trials that showed lifestyle interventions had a greater impact on diabetes prevention than medication, specifically metformin therapy. The USDPP assigned 3,234 participants age 25 to 85 years to a diet and exercise regimen, metformin, or a control group. The Da Qing China, Finnish Diabetes Prevention Study, and the Japanese Prevention Trials were smaller trials showing the effectiveness of lifestyle intervention.

156. A) Drug–drug interactions
This patient is at risk for drug–drug interactions, likely due to mismanaged polypharmacy. The patient reports confusion on medication schedules, which puts the patient even more at risk for negative outcomes. The majority of adverse events are correlated with the following medication classes: warfarin, insulins, oral antiplatelet agents, and hypoglycemic agents. Given the patient's history of a pulmonary embolism and diabetes, it is likely they are taking medications from most, if not all, of those medication classes. There is no information given in the patient's history or report to suggest they are having a drug-induced allergic reaction. It is more likely the patient would experience hypoglycemia with the combination of medication classes they are likely taking. The patient expresses difficulty with remembering their medication schedule, not an unwillingness to follow their schedule.

157. C) "Tell the counselor to immediately give the child four glucose tablets and recheck blood sugar in 15 minutes."

Instructing the counselor to give the child four glucose tablets immediately and recheck blood sugar in 15 minutes is following the "rule of 15." In this case, the counselor's error was in giving only one tablet, which most often equals 4 g of carbohydrates and is not enough to raise the blood glucose to a safe level. The camp staff, parents, and child would benefit from a review of the "rule of 15" and the nutrition facts and serving size on the label of the glucose tablets. The priority in this situation is treating the hypoglycemic episode; the type of activity the child was engaged in is irrelevant to the treatment protocol. This situation requires a quick response but does not necessitate calling 911 because the patient has not yet been properly treated. Waiting 30 minutes would result in the child's blood sugar decreasing further. The correct protocol is to wait 15 minutes after administering sufficient glucose.

158. D) Designate a diabetes resource nurse to provide an in-service and mentor peers on their units

Designating a diabetes resource nurse, or "champion," to help train and mentor the other staff would be the most ideal solution. This would ensure that there is always a staff member who is properly trained on insulin pumps. Webinars may be helpful, but hands-on and experiential learning with insulin pumps is more effective. Assigning patients who have insulin pumps to nurses who are already familiar with pumps may create an unequal burden on those nurses and deprive other staff from learning this important skill. Consulting a diabetes educator would be a good idea for any patients who are newly diagnosed, not maintaining good glycemic control, or struggling with their diabetes equipment or who could benefit from outpatient follow-up. However, it would benefit all nursing staff to have at least a basic understanding and working knowledge of a pump to be able to assist their patients if needed.

159. A) Aspirin

The ADA recommends 75 to 162 mg/d of aspirin for patients with diabetes and atherosclerotic cardiovascular disease to reduce risk of cardiovascular events. Insulin and metformin are used to reduce blood glucose levels. Simvastatin is used to treat elevated cholesterol and triglycerides.

160. C) "I will eat when my schedule allows."

Eating when your schedule allows with fixed/premixed insulins may cause hypoglycemia. Eating consistent carbohydrates that match the insulin dosing at regular intervals is the best way to stabilize the glucose and prevent hypoglycemia.

161. C) Taking the prescribed insulin postprandial
Taking insulin postprandial will cause spikes in postprandial glucose levels, since rapid-acting insulin takes 15 minutes to absorb into the tissue and then peaks at 1.5 to 2 hours. Taking insulin 15 to 20 minutes prior to meals can help alleviate postprandial spiking, as can proper insulin-to-carbohydrate-ratio dosing.

162. A) The patient is having postprandial spikes between 250 and 300 mg/dL
Postprandial spiking is likely the pattern causing an elevated A1C, despite the patient's glucose logs. The nocturnal glucose as well as the fasting and morning glucose could also be elevated but are not likely the cause of elevation in the A1C.

163. A) Educate the patient on a diet low in simple carbohydrates and reduce insulin by 50%
Educating the patient on a low-simple carbohydrate diet and reducing insulin by 50% (25% for the hypoglycemic reaction plus another 25% for the reduction in carbohydrates) is the best immediate intervention. Sitagliptin could also be added during this time but would require a larger insulin reduction to prevent hypoglycemia. A GLP-1 would benefit the patient eventually but if added now would require a larger insulin reduction. A lower-calorie diet might reduce carbohydrate intake but would require a larger insulin reduction as well.

164. B) Intradermal skin testing
The most effective diagnostic tool is an intradermal insulin skin test to confirm an insulin allergy. From this, the allergen can be identified, and then a review of the allergens common to all insulin excipients can be done to determine the type of insulin that can be used. A blood test, skin prick test, or patch test will not confirm the presence of allergens related to insulin.

165. B) How many times a day is the patient checking their glucose?
Knowing how many times per day the patient is actually testing glucose enables the clinician to set a realistic goal. It is appropriate to see if the patient has interest in a CGM but not before knowing whether the patient is testing regularly. Asking the patient why they aren't testing can put them on the defensive, setting a negative tone for motivating the patient. Involving the parents might be appropriate, but getting more information directly from the patient would be the priority in this intervention.

166. B) Have the patient check glucose levels before dinner and 2 hours postprandial

The most accurate assessment is to check the glucose level before the meal and then 2 hours postprandial. Premeal glucose is important data, as it reveals the specific increase in blood glucose postprandial. Data at 1, 2, or 3 hours postprandial alone shows the glucose at its highest and specific declined levels but lacks the premeal baseline needed for the full picture.

167. B) Fasting, before meals, bedtime, and 2 a.m.

Patients newly diagnosed and on insulin need to check when fasting to evaluate basal insulin dosing, before meals to determine mealtime insulin dosing, at bedtime to prevent hypoglycemia, and at 2 a.m. to prevent nocturnal hypoglycemia. Any other schedule would not be sufficient for safety and would offer insufficient data points for evaluation of insulin regimen.

168. A) Review survival skills verbally and have the patient repeat back the dosing instructions

Having the patient understand the risks of insulin is imperative prior to their going home. By using teach-back, the educator can verify patient understanding of the concepts. Writing the instructions down and verbally telling the patient do not guarantee understanding. The patient might have a family member or friend who could be included, but since the patient lives alone, it is important that they understand the regimen independently as well. A follow-up phone call can be helpful as well, but it is not enough combined with the instructions.

169. D) Advise the patient to continue with current lifestyle choices

Though the patient's LDL is greater than 100 mg/dL, their BP, A1C, and remaining lipids are within normal limits. The patient is meeting goals for exercise as well. Reduction of fat intake may not necessarily help with lowering LDL, but it could be reduced by increasing dietary fiber. A statin would only be advised based on the patient's cardiovascular risks or overt cardiovascular disease.

170. C) The patient can take insulin 30 minutes before breakfast and dinner

The patient must take the insulin 30 minutes before breakfast and dinner, since the regular insulin takes 30 to 45 minutes for onset, and the NPH insulin has a duration of 1 to 2 hours. Splitting these meals by 12 hours is optimal. This insulin should not be given more than twice daily due to the action of the NPH. Verifying the accuracy of the prescription directions is important, as it may be inconsistent with the instructions given by the provider.

171. D) A1C to be less than 8% within 3 months

For an 80-year-old patient with comorbidities, an A1C of 8% is a realistic goal. Weighing the risks versus the benefits is important given the patient's age and complex medical history. Attempting to get the patient to an A1C of <7% might induce hypoglycemia and present the patient with undue stress. An exercise program might be appropriate if it would not put stress on the patient's heart and was approved by their cardiologist. Postprandial goals of <180 mg/dL might be too restrictive for this patient as well.

172. D) Pattern management

Pattern management is a systematic approach that allows SMBG data to be viewed by both the patient and the provider to identify patterns that allow for optimizing control of blood glucose. This is an advanced SMBG education topic that would be an appropriate next area to discuss. Finger site selection and hypoglycemia and hyperglycemia definitions are basic concepts of SMBG. The patient already has a basic and intermediate understanding of SMBG. How the chemicals in the strip react with glucose is an advanced concept but is not considered need-to-know information that can help the patient practically self-manage their disease.

173. C) Avoid exposing insulin to temperatures above 86°F

The most critical educational goal is teaching the patient that their insulin should be kept at less than 86°F. Providing the patient with a cooling pack in this case could be an intervention. Insulin should be kept in the dark as sunlight breaks down insulin, insulin can be stored at room temperature after it has been opened, and unused insulin should be kept at 36°F to 46°F; however, none of these are the most imperative educational goal for the patient.

174. A) Inquire about the patient's level of understanding and what they want to learn

One of the most effective strategies for assessment of learning needs is to ask patients about their level of understanding of their condition and treatment and what they want to learn. Asking how long they have had diabetes would not be effective because the patient's duration of disease does not always correlate with their learning needs. The PHQ-9 questionnaire is a screening tool to help identify depression, not overall learning needs. Including family members and caregivers in the discussion may be appropriate for some patients, but not all patients want to include other family members in their planning process.

175. B) Fifth to sixth grade

It is recommended to use materials written at a fifth- to sixth-grade reading level. It is estimated that about one third of Americans have low health literacy. Material written at a twelfth-grade level or higher is above the level of understanding of many patients with diabetes. Material written at a second- to third-grade level is below the recommended reading level and would oversimplify important topics. Customizing materials for each patient depending on their reading level would provide tailored education to all patients but is not a practical approach because materials must be developed in advance, must be cost effective, and are often provided to patients in group settings.

176. B) How often the patient currently performs SMBG

The provider should inquire how often the patient is performing SMBG. Obtaining a baseline for diabetes self-management allows for setting realistic and measurable goals that are attainable in a short period of time. Knowing the patient's meal and activity schedule, most recent A1C, and the members of their support network would help pinpoint times to perform SMBG, determine current glycemic control, and identify sources of support to achieve goals, respectively, but this information does not provide a baseline of the patient's diabetes self-management.

177. D) Provide scenarios of meals and premeal blood glucose values and ask the parents to calculate proper insulin doses

Providing multiple scenarios of different meals and snacks, including carbohydrate content, and different premeal blood glucose values and asking the parents to calculate the proper insulin doses is the most effective way to help them learn. Effective educational strategies include involving patients or family members in the patient's care and guiding them in actively learning about the disease by providing fewer topics and more practice. The 1800 rule is a way for healthcare providers to calculate the carbohydrate ratio and sensitivity factor to prescribe to a patient and is not a topic that the parents need to understand. How to test the carbohydrate ratio is a more advanced topic that should be addressed only after the parents have learned how to calculate insulin doses. Providing written materials that explain the concepts of carbohydrate ratio and insulin sensitivity factor may be helpful but does not allow the parents to practice calculating doses or the diabetes educator to assess their level of understanding.

178. C) When glucose levels are rising or falling rapidly
A patient is more likely to see significant differences between CGM measures of interstitial glucose and plasma glucose when glucose levels are rising or falling rapidly. This is due to a lag time between the interstitial glucose and the plasma glucose. When glucose levels are rising rapidly, the CGM reading will be lower than the plasma glucose. When glucose levels are falling rapidly, the CGM reading will be higher than the plasma glucose. The sensor should be accurate until it has expired and is often more accurate after several days of wear than it is on the first and second day of use. Sensors are approved to be worn on the back of the arm, and placement here does not affect differences any more than placement at other approved sites.

179. D) Rapid-acting insulin
Rapid-acting insulin is delivered through insulin pump therapy. Insulin pumps deliver rapid-acting insulin continuously throughout the day, known as basal insulin, and boluses of rapid acting-insulin when the patient consumes carbohydrates, performs a correction, or both. Rapid-acting insulin is used for both basal and bolus coverage.

180. B) The patient should be instructed to pre-bolus before meals
The patient should be instructed to pre-bolus before meals. A pattern of hyperglycemia followed by hypoglycemia with meals indicates that the patient is not pre-bolusing or taking insulin prior to the meal with enough time to match the insulin's peak action with the meal digestion time. Strengthening the carbohydrate ratio would be appropriate if the patient had sustained hyperglycemia following the meal without hypoglycemia. Increasing the basal rate prior to the meal and then decreasing it after the meal would not compensate for the sharp rise in blood sugar due to lack of pre-bolusing and hypoglycemia that occurs afterward. Strengthening the sensitivity factor is indicated when it is noted that the patient gives a correction, but the blood sugar fails to return to the patient's baseline within 4 to 5 hours.

181. C) Low self-efficacy
The patient is exhibiting low self-efficacy. Self-efficacy is the belief in one's ability to succeed in a specific situation. Even when a patient understands the importance of changing a behavior, changing the behavior is difficult without self-efficacy. Low motivation is also a barrier, but this patient states that they want to improve their health, demonstrating proper motivation. Numeracy includes calculations and quantitative skills; the patient has not expressed concerns around this issue. Noncompliance means not following a healthcare provider's recommendations. There are many reasons for noncompliance, including low self-efficacy and low motivation, but noncompliance is the result of these barriers, not the barrier itself.

182. C) Diabetes distress

Diabetes distress is used to describe a sense of being overwhelmed or a feeling of failure or frustration developed by an individual with diabetes. This is different from depression, anxiety, and denial because it is specific to diabetes. Denial, depression, and anxiety may also apply to individuals who do not have diabetes.

183. A) Numeracy

The patient may have problems with numeracy. Numeracy skills involve calculations or other quantitative skills that are required to function in the healthcare system. The physician has given medication instructions, but the patient lacks an understanding of how to incorporate their sensitivity factor when calculating insulin doses. Diabetes distress refers to negative psychologic reactions related to the burden of managing a chronic disease, which the patient is not exhibiting. Not being able to recall their sensitivity factor, rather than not using their sensitivity factor, would suggest a memory problem. Reading literacy is not a factor because the patient has not been provided with written materials.

184. D) Action

The patient is in the action stage as evidenced by the overt behavior changes they have made. The patient is not in the maintenance stage because they have not sustained the behavior changes for 6 months or longer. The patient is not in the preparation stage because they have already made overt behavior changes. The patient is not in the contemplation stage because they have already taken action.

185. B) Precontemplation, contemplation, preparation, action, and maintenance

Precontemplation, contemplation, preparation, action, and maintenance are the five stages included in the transtheoretical model of change. In the precontemplation stage, the patient is not intending to change in the foreseeable future. In the contemplation stage, the patient is not prepared to take action at present but is intending to within the next 6 months. In the preparation stage, the patient is actively considering changing their behavior in the immediate future. In the action stage, the patient has made a behavior change in the recent past, but the changes are not well established. In the maintenance stage, the patient has changed their behavior for longer than 6 months and is working to sustain the change. Termination is sometimes included but is less often used in the application of stages for health-related behaviors. Revision, skills acquisition, and self-evaluation are not included in the transtheoretical model of change.

186. D) Provide one-on-one education

This patient is in the precontemplation stage, during which the individual is not intending to change in the foreseeable future. When this stage is identified, the patient responds better to individually tailored interventions and should meet with a diabetes educator one on one. Cognitive capacity should be monitored for this patient at some point, but this is more of a priority for patients with documented cognitive disabilities, those who experience severe hypoglycemia, very young children, and older adults. Referral to an endocrinologist would not be helpful until the patient was willing to accept and follow a treatment plan. Providing continuous glucose monitoring training would be more appropriate for a patient who accepts their diagnosis but does not like performing finger sticks.

187. A) Discuss relative hypoglycemia

It is most important to discuss relative hypoglycemia with this patient. The provider should acknowledge their symptoms but also discuss glucose targets and treatment goals and educate the patient that symptoms of relative hypoglycemia will improve once blood sugars have normalized. The rule of 15 is important to address with all patients on insulin but should not be implemented unless the blood sugar is less than 70 mg/dL. A bedtime snack would only be recommended if the patient was having true hypoglycemia. Hypoglycemia unawareness is a complication of diabetes in which patients are unaware of hypoglycemia, which is not an issue for this patient.

188. B) Glucagon

Glucagon is released by the liver following untreated hypoglycemia. Amylin is a hormone that suppresses appetite and slows stomach movements, preventing hyperglycemia after meals. Incretin hormones help release insulin and delay the release of glucose, resulting in euglycemia rather than hyperglycemia. Insulin promotes glucose uptake in the cells, which may cause euglycemia or hypoglycemia but not hyperglycemia.

189. A) Ask the patient what they need from family members regarding their diabetes management

The patient should be given the opportunity to voice what they need from family members regarding their diabetes management. This gives the family a direction on how to support their child but avoids miscarried helping. At this age, the patient can manage many aspects of diabetes self-care independently but benefits from support in order to distribute the burdens of diabetes management. Encouraging the patient to self-manage their diabetes independently is inappropriate because it does not distribute the burdens of diabetes management. Prescribing a continuous glucose monitoring device that allows data sharing does not provide the patient an opportunity to voice their needs and may not be in their interest. Educating the patient and the family members about the complications that can result from worsening control only highlights the problem and does not allow the patient and their family to come to a solution that meets the patient's needs.

190. C) Educate the patient on the direct and indirect effects of alcohol on blood glucose levels

The patient should be educated on the direct and indirect effects of alcohol on blood glucose levels. Although the carbohydrates in some alcoholic beverages may raise blood sugar, alcohol can also cause hypoglycemia due to inhibition of gluconeogenesis. Advising the patient to abstain from alcohol is not the best response because the recommendations for consuming alcoholic beverages are the same for people with and without diabetes. Telling the patient to take rapid-acting insulin prior to drinking to cover the carbohydrates in alcoholic beverages could result in hypoglycemia. Ensuring that the patient has a prescription for glucagon (e.g., Glucagon Emergency Kit, Baqsimi) is inappropriate because the liver is unable to break down glycogen when detoxing the body of alcohol, rendering the administration of glucagon useless.

191. A) Sulfonylureas

Sulfonylureas may cause hypoglycemia because they stimulate the pancreatic beta cells to secrete insulin. This risk is heightened when they are consumed with alcohol due to its effect on the inhibition of gluconeogenesis. Thiazolidinediones, biguanides, and SGLT2 inhibitors do not have a higher risk of hypoglycemia when paired with alcohol because these medications do not stimulate the release of insulin.

192. A) Review the patient's current self-care skills

Reviewing the patient's current self-care skills is a good place to start. Once the medical team, the patient, and the family agree on where the patient's skills are, goals for achieving increased skills should be discussed and agreed upon. Encouraging the patient to begin independently managing their diabetes as soon as possible is not necessary at this age when the patient is likely to achieve greater confidence in their self-care skills with additional support. Transferring the patient to an adult provider usually occurs between the ages of 18 and 21 years. Having the patient attend healthcare appointments independently is inappropriate because parents should still be aware of changes in the plan of care. However, many pediatricians will begin to spend a few minutes alone with their patients at this stage, giving them the experience of talking directly with their provider and helping them develop communication and self-advocacy skills.

193. B) Refer them to a behavioral health provider

Patients should be referred to a mental healthcare provider when self-care remains impaired in a person with diabetes distress after tailored diabetes education. Group therapy would not address diabetes distress adequately or be tailored to the patient. Reviewing the complications of uncontrolled diabetes is not necessary because the diabetes educator would have already made sure the patient was aware of these complications. Prescribing mixed insulin twice a day to reduce the number of injections the patient needs to take is inappropriate because mixed insulin is not a recommended treatment for people with type 1 diabetes.

194. D) Cognitive capacity

The provider should assess the patient's cognitive capacity. Episodes of severe hypoglycemia are associated with cognitive decline, and it is important to ascertain the patient's ability to manage their diabetes and perform self-care practices such as taking and dosing medications and treating hypoglycemia. Injuries from falls would be important to assess only if the hypoglycemic events happened recently. The patient does not report symptoms of depression, which include feelings of sadness, hopelessness, and loss of interest in activities. Assessing adherence to medications is inappropriate because lack of adherence would cause hyperglycemia, not hypoglycemia.

195. B) Decline in beta-cell function
A decline in beta-cell function is responsible for the change in the patient's condition. A progressive decline in beta-cell function over several years, regardless of therapy, was demonstrated in the U.K. Prospective Diabetes Study. With significant decline, patients are not able to produce enough of their own insulin to control blood sugar levels and will require insulin therapy. According to the same study, insulin resistance does not change, and blood sugars still respond to oral medications when resistance is present. Autoimmunity is present in type 1 diabetes, not type 2 diabetes. Decreased incretin effect is present in type 2 diabetes but can be treated with noninsulin therapy.

196. D) They should not go 2 or more consecutive days without activity
The patient should not go 2 or more consecutive days without activity. According to the 2022 American Diabetes Association Standards of Medical Care, most adults with diabetes should engage in 150 minutes of moderate- to vigorous-intensity aerobic activity, spread over at least 3 days per week, with no more than 2 consecutive days without activity. They do not need to add 30 to 60 minutes of activity because they are already engaging in more than 150 minutes of activity. Many patients are able to exercise 2 or more days in a row without causing injury. The patient does not need to add resistance training during the week because they are already meeting the recommended goal of two to three sessions of resistance training per week.

197. B) Information about consistent patterns of carbohydrate intake
Information about consistent patterns of carbohydrate intake is the most important education to provide to this patient. Patients on fixed mealtime insulin doses need to eat a consistent amount of carbohydrates for their insulin to work effectively. This patient is reporting meals that are highly variable in carbohydrate amounts that will cause hyperglycemia and hypoglycemia. Although low-carbohydrate diets have demonstrated the most evidence for improving glycemia, this would not be an appropriate educational topic for a patient on fixed mealtime insulin doses. A Mediterranean-style eating pattern is beneficial to improve glucose metabolism and lower cardiovascular disease, but it does not emphasize carbohydrate consistency. Education on the glycemic impact of carbohydrates, fats, and proteins is more beneficial to a patient on flexible insulin therapy, not fixed doses.

198. C) They should schedule a consultation with an ophthalmologist

The patient should schedule a consultation with an ophthalmologist prior to starting weight training. Patients with nonproliferative diabetic retinopathy or proliferative diabetic retinopathy should consult an ophthalmologist prior to engaging in vigorous-intensity aerobic or resistance exercise due to the risk of triggering vitreous hemorrhage or retinal detachment. Adults with diabetes should try to engage in two to three sessions of resistance training a week on nonconsecutive days, but this may be contraindicated for this patient. Flexibility training and balance training two to three times per week is recommended for older adults with diabetes, but this does not address the patient's risk of triggering vitreous hemorrhage or retinal detachment. Referral to cardiology would not be indicated for proliferative diabetic retinopathy without other complications.

199. D) Quinolones

Quinolones (a type of antibiotic) can cause glucose levels to drop, whereas glucocorticoids, thiazide diuretics, and atypical antipsychotics (clozapine, olanzapine, and risperidone) can cause glucose levels to rise.

200. A) Age, duration of symptoms, and glucose levels

When comparing DKA and HHS, the biggest differences are in age, duration of symptoms, glucose levels, bicarbonate levels, and presence of ketone bodies. Similarities can exist in sodium and potassium concentration.